TRANSMITTERS IN THE VISUAL PROCESS

Other Pergamon Press Titles of Interest

USDIN and SNYDER	*Frontiers in Catecholamine Research*
USDIN et al	*Catecholamines and Stress*

TRANSMITTERS IN THE VISUAL PROCESS

Edited by

S.L. Bonting, Ph.D.

Department of Biochemistry
University of Nijmegen

PERGAMON PRESS

OXFORD · NEW YORK · TORONTO · SYDNEY · PARIS · FRANKFURT

U.K. Pergamon Press Ltd., Headington Hill Hall, Oxford OX3 0BW, England

U.S.A. Pergamon Press Inc., Maxwell House, Fairview Park, Elmsford, New York 10523, U.S.A.

CANADA Pergamon of Canada Ltd., P.O. Box 9600, Don Mills M3C 2T9, Ontario, Canada

AUSTRALIA Pergamon Press (Aust.) Pty. Ltd., 19a Boundary Street, Rushcutters Bay, N.S.W. 2011, Australia

FRANCE Pergamon Press SARL, 24 rue des Ecoles, 75240 Paris, Cedex 05, France

WEST GERMANY Pergamon Press GmbH, 6242 Kronberg-Taunus, Pferdstrasse 1, Frankfurt-am-Main, West Germany

---

First edition 1976

Library of Congress Cataloging in Publication Data

Main entry under title:

Transmitters in the visual process.

Consists of expanded versions of papers presented at a symposium held at the fifth international meeting of the International Society for Neurochemistry, in Barcelona, Spain in September 1975.
Includes index.
1. Vision--Congresses. 2. Neural transmission-- Congresses.
3. Retina--Innervation--Congresses.
I. Bonting, Sjoerd Lieuwe. II. International Society for Neurochemistry. [DNLM:
1. Neural transmission--Congresses. 2. Vision--Congresses.
3. Photoreceptors--Physiology--Congresses. 4. Retina--Physiology--Congresses.
WW103 T772 1975]
QP474.T7 1976 612'.84 76-5159
ISBN 0-08-020907-6

In order to make this volume available as economically and rapidly as possible the author's typescript has been reproduced in its original form. This method unfortunately has its typographical limitations but it is hoped that they in no way distract the reader.

Printed in Great Britain by A. Wheaton & Co. Exeter

CONTENTS

PREFACE

This book is the result of a symposium under the same title, held at the Fifth International Meeting of the International Society for Neurochemistry in Barcelona, Spain in September, 1975.

The usefulness of symposium books, particularly those giving little more than a series of individual papers and often appearing after a long delay, can be questioned. Most of the material has by then also appeared in journals, or is about to appear, often with somewhat different conclusions because the authors were led to bring their latest, but not yet fully tested findings at the symposium. This then results in a confusing situation for the less initiated students of the literature in the field.

In organizing the present symposium it became clear to the editor that a somewhat different situation exists. The subject has been receiving widespread attention only in recent years, so that no books and only one or two reviews have appeared. Secondly, it is a multidisciplinary field frequented by visual scientists with little previous experience of transmitter physiology and pharmacology as well as by transmitter experts who know little about the visual system. Thirdly, it affords an interesting opportunity of considering together with the synaptic transmitters the intracellular transmitters, like the cyclic nucleotides and calcium ions, which appear to have much in common with the former substances in their mode of action.

In order to make this book more useful the authors have been asked to expand their symposium presentations so as to offer an adequate review of the literature on their topic, to describe the techniques used and to indicate the questions remaining unanswered. Two additional papers (ch. 8 and 9) have been invited for this book, which complement the others. It is regretted that the coverage of the optic tract is rather brief, but this probably reflects the rudimentary state of our knowledge of this aspect.

It is hoped that the resulting book will be useful to all workers in this field, as well as to those about to enter it, and that it may stimulate the research on transmitters in the visual system in the next several years.

The editor wishes to acknowledge the excellent cooperation received from the authors as well as from the publishers, and he particularly wants to thank his secretary, Mrs. T. Hinlopen-Kassies, for her expert care in preparing the manuscript.

S.L. Bonting

CHAPTER 1

STRUCTURE AND MECHANISM OF THE VERTEBRATE VISUAL SYSTEM

S.L. Bonting

Dept. of Biochemistry
University of Nijmegen
Nijmegen, The Netherlands

INTRODUCTION

The visual system consists of a rather complicated network of various types of cells, which function in transmitting the signal of a photon absorbed in a photoreceptor cell to the brain. A proper integration of light signals from a number of photoreceptor cells into an image requires the coupling of different cells to each other. Such junctions, called synapses, are well known in the nervous system. In synapses between two nerve cells the signal crosses the gap between the two interconnected cells by releasing a chemical transmitter substance from the terminal of the presynaptic neuron. The transmitter substance then excites the postsynaptic neuron, where an electric impulse is generated and carried along to its terminal (see e.g.: Bachelard, 1974, pp 18-41). Instead of exciting the postsynaptic neuron, the transmitter may also inhibit its electric activity. The conventional synapse in the nervous system and its mechanism are shown schematically in Fig. 1.1. In the retina we find not only this conventional synapse, but also two other kinds: the ribbon type and the flat contact type, which will be described further down. These synapses probably all rely on transmitter substances for the transmission of the signal. In addition, there is a type of synapse, which does not make use of a transmitter, the electric synapse or gap junction. This is a region of low resistance through which current can pass from one cell to the other. It is formed by the close apposition of the membranes of the two adjacent cells, leaving a narrow gap containing a lattice of polygonal subunits.

Inside the rod photoreceptor cell we also find a situation, where an impulse must cross a gap between two membranes: from the rod sac membrane to the outer membrane of the rod outer segment. There is reason to assume that in this instance also a transmitter substance is involved. This substance would be released from the rod sacs after the absorption of a photon by the visual pigment present in the rod sac membrane. Such a substance we shall call an intracellular transmitter to distinguish it from the synaptic transmitters.

It is the purpose of this Symposium to survey our present knowledge and current findings about synaptic and intracellular transmitters in the visual

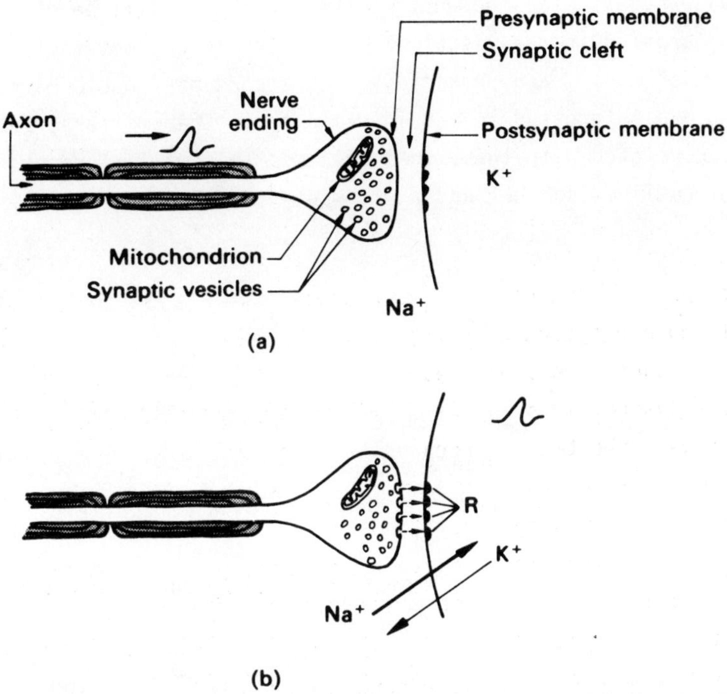

Fig. 1.1. Schematic presentation of synaptic transmission. On arrival of the action potential at the nerve ending (a), transmitter molecules are released and react with receptors (R) on the post-synaptic membrane. This leads to a change in ion permeability of this membrane (b). After Bachelard (1974).

system. The synaptic transmitters in this system have previously been reviewed by Graham (1974). Questions to be discussed in this context are: the identity, the localization and the mechanism of the transmitter. The complex structure of the retina and optical tract as well as the minute quantities of transmitter operating in a very small region pose severe methodological problems, which will also be considered.

In this introductory chapter we shall first describe the criteria to be met in order to classify a substance as a transmitter and the main types of transmitters known today. Thereafter, we shall briefly outline the structure of the vertebrate visual system and our current insight in the mechanism of the visual process. It is hoped that the first part will be of help to persons interested in the visual process, but who are not familiar with transmitter chemistry and physiology. The second part would have to assist those, who are interested in and informed about transmitters, but who are not well acquainted with the visual process. This will of necessity have to be a brief outline, so the reader who wants to delve deeper will be referred to recent books and reviews in these fields.

SYNAPTIC AND INTRACELLULAR TRANSMITTERS

Criteria for a transmitter

From the early experience with acetylcholine (Dale et al., 1936) five criteria, which can be used to assess whether a substance qualifies as a synaptic transmitter, have been formulated:

1. The substance must be synthesized and/or stored in the nerve endings from which it is released.
2. The substance must be released upon pre-synaptic stimulation and shown to be present in the extracellular fluid in the vicinity.
3. When applied post-synaptically it must mimic the action seen when the pre-synaptic system is stimulated.
4. Specific antagonists should be able to block both the natural transmission and the action of the substance. Such antagonists usually block the interaction of the transmitter with its receptor on the post-synaptic membrane.
5. There must be a mechanism for the removal of the transmitter from the post-synaptic region, either by chemical transformation, diffusion or re-uptake in the pre-synaptic nerve ending.

The classical work of Dale and co-workers (Dale, 1935; Dale et al., 1936; Brown et al., 1936) on the neuromuscular junction demonstrated that acetylcholine satisfies criteria 2 - 5. Application of the substance mimicks the effect of stimulating parasympathetic nerves. Stimulation of the vagus nerve causes release of acetylcholine. Curare blocks both the effect of stimulation and of acetylcholine application. The enzyme acetylcholinesterase hydrolyses the released acetylcholine, and inhibitors of the enzyme, like physostigmine, potentiate nerve stimulation. The first criterion was shown to be satisfied some thirty years later, when the isolation of nerve endings was accomplished simultaneously by Whittaker (Gray and Whittaker, 1962) and De Robertis et al.

(1962) through centrifugal fractionation of brain homogenates. Gentle homogenization breaks the axon near the point where it widens into the nerve ending. The broken membrane generally re-seals to produce an ending which is intact and is called a "synaptosome" (Marchbanks and Whittaker, 1969). Analysis showed that the synaptosomes have a high acetylcholine concentration and are also high in the enzymes required for its synthesis.

For intracellular transmitters a similar set of five criteria can be formulated. They are synthesized by a specific enzyme, in the case of cyclic AMP by a membrane-bound cyclase, or stored in an intracellular structure, e.g. the sarcoplasmic reticulum in the case of calcium in the muscle. They are released upon stimulation, e.g. hormones release cyclic AMP and stimulation of the neuromuscular junction releases calcium ions from the sarcoplasmic reticulum. Upon exogenous application to the target membrane, the substance must mimic the action seen after stimulation of the intracellular structure. This has in many cases been shown for the cyclic nucleotides and in some cases also for calcium ions. Specific antagonists, which act similarly on the effect of stimulation and of adding the transmitter, are not known in the case of the cyclic nucleotides, while for calcium a binding agent like EGTA might be cited. Finally, there must be a mechanism for removal of the released transmitter from the target membrane and the cytoplasm. For the cyclic nucleotides this is the phosphodiesterase, which converts them to inactive substances. Calcium is generally removed by reaccumulation in the storage structure.

Classes of transmitters

Since the discovery of acetylcholine many other synaptic transmitters have been recognized in the vertebrate system. The various classes of synaptic and intracellular transmitters are listed, where possible together with their antagonists, in Table 1.

Their location has been determined in various ways: by chemical analysis of tissues and parts of tissues, by isolation and analysis of synaptosomes and by histochemical techniques. A very useful histochemical technique has been fluorescence microscopy after exposure of frozen or freeze-dried sections to formaldehyde vapour. Catecholamines give blue-green (470 nm) and serotonin yellow (520 nm) fluorescence (Falck, 1962). Radioautographic methods have

Table 1.1. Proven and alleged transmitters in vertebrates

Name	Structure	Antagonists
A. Synaptic transmitters		
1. Acetylcholine	$CH_3COOCH_2CH_2\overset{+}{N}(CH_3)_3$	Curare; atropine
2. Catecholamines		
a) Noradrenaline	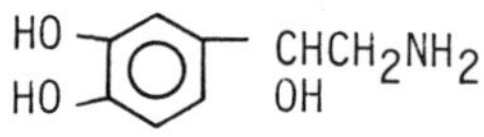	Ergot alkaloids (α-blocker) Propanolol (β-blocker)
b) Dopamine	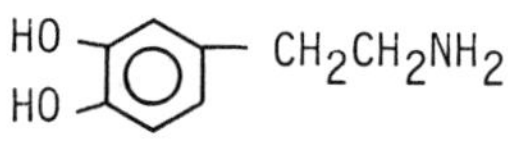	Haloperidol Spiroperidol
3. Serotonin	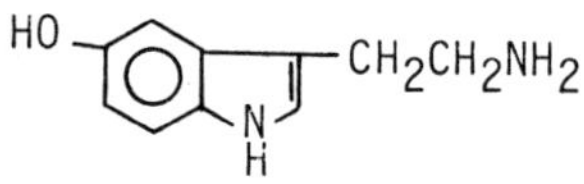	Methergoline, LSD
4. Amino acids		
a) Glycine	$HOOCCH_2NH_2$	Strychnine
b) γAminobutyrate (GABA)	$HOOCCH_2CH_2CH_2NH_2$	Bicuculline Picrotoxin Benzylpenicillin
c) Taurine	$HO_3SCH_2CH_2NH_2$	Strychnine
d) Glutamate	$HOOCCHNH_2$ CH_2CH_2COOH	-
e) Aspartate	$HOOCCHNH_2$ CH_2COOH	-
f) Proline	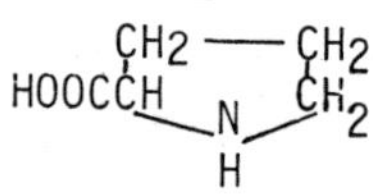	-
B. Intracellular transmitters		
1. Cyclic AMP	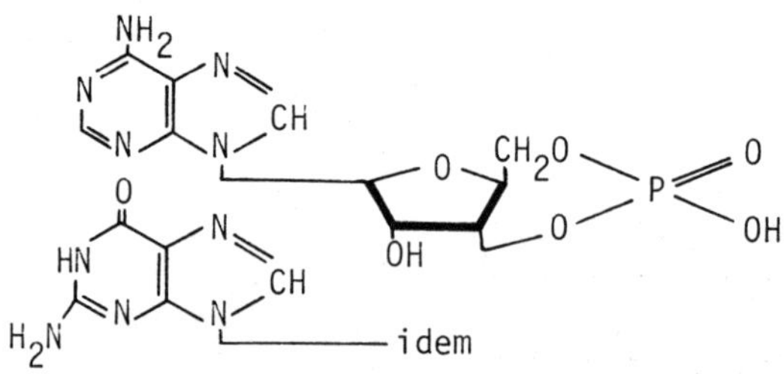	-
2. Cyclic GMP		-
3. Calcium ions		-

also been of great help. An important technique for identifying a substance as a transmitter is to apply it locally through one channel of a multi-barreled micropipette electrode by means of iontophoresis and monitor its effects electrophysiologically through another channel of the electrode (Curtis, 1964).

The metabolism, synthesis as well as catabolism of these transmitters has been studied extensively. The results can be found in most textbooks of biochemistry and neurochemistry (e.g. White, Handler and Smith, 1973; Lajtha, 1969-73). Acetylcholine is very efficiently hydrolyzed by acetylcholinesterase. The catecholamines and serotonin can be inactivated by monoamine oxidase, which is present in neurones; the catecholamines can also be inactivated extraneuronally by the enzyme catechol-O-methyltransferase. However, the main mechanism for the inactivation of the latter transmitters appears to be re-uptake into the neurone.

Two types of effects of synaptic transmitters can be distinguished on the basis of their postsynaptic action. Transmitters are excitatory, when they increase the permeability of the postsynaptic membrane preferentially to sodium ions, thereby depolarizing it, and thus causing excitation of the affected neurone. Transmitters are inhibitory, when they increase the permeability to chloride and possibly to potassium of the postsynaptic membrane, thereby hyperpolarizing it, and thus causing inhibition of the affected neurone. The amino acid transmitters are usually, but not always, inhibitory (review: Curtis and Johnston, 1973), while acetylcholine and the catecholamines are usually excitatory. Ultimately, the receptor on the postsynaptic membrane appears to determine, whether the transmitter effect will be excitatory or inhibitory.

The intracellular transmitters have, of course, an entirely different mechanism of action. The cyclic nucleotide 3'5' adenosine monophosphate (cyclic AMP) is believed to transmit the effect of a hormone or neurohumoral agent to an intracellular system (see e.g. Robison et al., 1971). Cyclic AMP is produced from ATP by the enzyme adenylate cyclase, which is located in the membrane. The enzyme consists of a hormone receptor on the outer face of the membrane and of a catalytic site on the inner face. Occupation of the receptor by the appropriate hormone activates the catalytic site. The resulting cyclic AMP enters the cytoplasm, where it may activate a protein kinase which stimulates through phosphorylation the target system (Langhan, 1973). It has been suggested that in the vertebrate peripheral nervous system catecholamine-stimulated production of cyclic AMP could lead to phosphorylation of membrane proteins resulting in hyperpolarisation of the postsynaptic membrane (Greengard and Kebabian, 1974).

Another cyclic nucleotide, 3',5' guanosinemonophosphate (cyclic GMP) may also act as a transmitter, since its concentration in several tissues is found to be increased by cholinergic agents, and this increase can be blocked by atropine (Goldberg et al., 1973). However, in this case no direct stimulation of a guanylcyclase by acetylcholine has been found, and there is evidence that the changes in cyclic GMP are regulated by changes in calcium concentration (Schultz et al., 1973). In various systems cyclic AMP and cyclic GMP behave antagonistically, increases of the one nucleotide often being accompanied by decreases of the other. This observation has been stressed by Goldberg et al. (1973) in the so-called Yin-Yang hypothesis. Since there are also cGMP-dependent protein kinases present in most tissues, the further mechanism of cyclic GMP might be analogous to that of cyclic AMP. The role of cyclic nucleotides in the visual system is discussed in detail in ch. 2 by Goridis et al., and in other context by Wassenaar and Korf in ch. 9.

Calcium ions have been shown to act as transmitter in various important cellular processes, like muscle contraction (see e.g. Fuchs, 1974) and secretion of enzymes by the pancreas (see e.g. Thorn and Petersen, 1974). Common feature of these processes is that in the resting state the cytoplasmic calcium ion concentration is extremely low (10^{-7}-10^{-6}M), while calcium is accumulated in very high concentration in an intracellular structure (sarcoplasmic reticulum in muscle, mitochondria in nerve, pancreas and salivary gland). Stimulation leads to release of calcium ions from the store, which increases the cytoplasmic calcium concentration and then leads to the desired effect. Thereafter, an efficient accumulation system must return the calcium ions again to the intracellular store. Such a role for calcium ions in the photoreceptor cell is discussed in chapter 3 by Bonting and Daemen.

STRUCTURE OF THE VERTEBRATE VISUAL SYSTEM

The structure of the vertebrate visual system will be described briefly with special emphasis on the synaptic relationships among the various cell types. This will be a qualitative description, largely ignoring quantitative and other differences between species. For a more extensive treatment of the subject the reader is referred to some recent books and reviews (Dowling, 1970; Stell, 1972; Dubin, 1974; Rodieck, 1973) and the classical treatise of Cajal, which is available in English translation as a monograph (Cajal, 1972) and as an appendix in the book of Rodieck (1973, pp 775-904).

Retinal layers

In the light microscope a fixed and stained section of the retina gives the appearance of a layered structure with seven main layers. These layers, going from pigment epithelium to vitreous, are called: 1. photoreceptor layer (PRL), 2. outer nuclear layer (ONL), 3. outer plexiform layer (OPL), 4. inner nuclear layer (INL), 5. inner plexiform layer (IPL), 6. ganglion cell layer (GCL), and 7. optic fiber layer (OFL). Application of special staining techniques, esp. the Golgi silver stain (Cajal, 1972), allowed to distinguish the various cell types arranged in such a way as to give the appearance of the seven-layer pattern. In recent years electron-microscopic studies, often coupled with electrophysiological observations, have further elucidated the types of cells and their interconnections.

The emerging picture is presented schematically in Fig. 1.2. The five principal cell types are:

1. photoreceptor cells, rods (R) and cones (C)
2. bipolar cells, midget type (MB), flat type (FB), rod bipolar (RB)
3. horizontal cells (H)
4. amacrine cells (A)
5. ganglion cells, midget (or tufted) type (MG), diffuse (or radiate) type (DG).

In addition there are the large Müller cells (glial cells), which extend vertically through the retina and which have fine processes that envelop all the nearby neurons. Their nuclei are located in the inner nuclear layer.

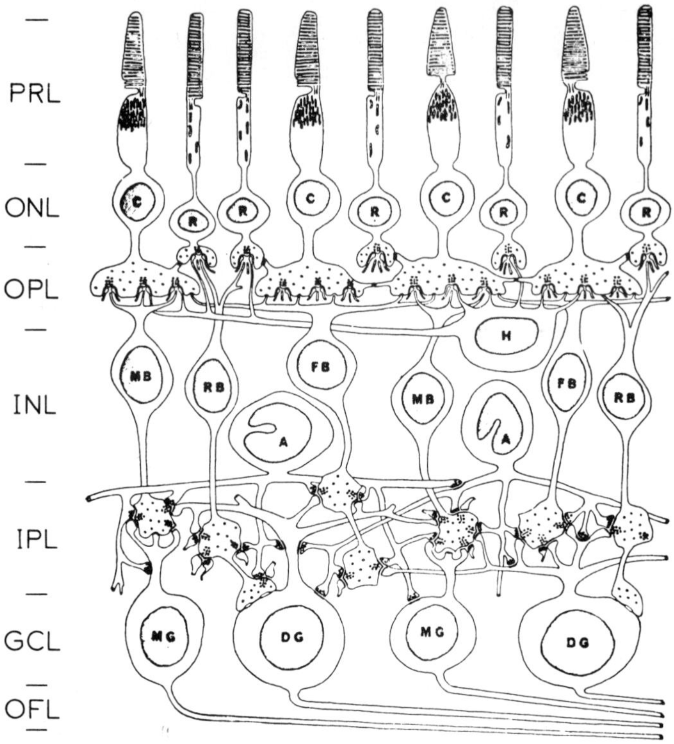

Fig. 1.2. Synaptic connections of the vertebrate retina (rhesus monkey and man). R, rod; C, cone; MB, midget bipolar, probably receiving only from one cone; FB, flat bipolar, receiving from several cones, but probably not from rods; RB, rod bipolar, receiving from several rods, but probably not from cones; H, horizontal cell; A, amacrine cell; MG, midget ganglion cell; DG, diffuse ganglion cell. On the left the retinal layers seen in light microscopy are indicated. PRL, photoreceptor layer, ONL, outer nuclear layer; OPL, outer plexiform layer, INL, inner nuclear layer; IPL, inner plexiform layer, GCL, ganglion cell layer; OFL, optic fiber layer. After Dowling, 1970.

The outer segment and distal part of the inner segment of the rods and cones form the photoreceptor layer (PRL). The nuclei of the rods and cones form the outer nuclear layer (ONL), while their synaptic endings form the outer plexiform layer (OPL). The cell bodies and nuclei of bipolar, horizontal and amacrine cells form the inner nuclear layer (INL), while the synapses between bipolar, amacrine and ganglion cells form the inner plexiform layer (IPL). The cell bodies and nuclei of the ganglion cells form the ganglion cell layer (GCL), and the axons of the ganglion cells, continuing into the optic nerve, form the optic fiber layer (OFL).

Very recently a new type of cell, an interplexiform neuron with the cell body located in the amacrine cell layer and with dendrites extending into both plexiform layers, has been demonstrated (Dowling and Ehinger, 1975). It appears to provide a centrifugal pathway from the inner to the outer plexiform layer.

Straight-through pathways

The interconnections between these cell types form two major types of pathways: the straight-through and the lateral pathways. The straight-through or three-neuron pathways consist of the route photoreceptor cell ⇒ bipolar cell ⇒ ganglion cell. Except for the midget bipolar cells (MB), which appear to connect with a single cone, the connections are multiple. The flat bipolar cell (FB) receives from several cones (but no rods), while the rod bipolar cell (RB) receives from several rods (but no cones). Conversely, individual photoreceptor cells usually make synapses with several bipolar cells. In Fig. 1.3 a schematic representation of the synapses of a rod and a cone are shown.

Some variations on the straight-through pathways just described have been noted. In certain fishes connections of both rods and cones to the same bipolar cell have been observed. In lower vertebrates, such as the frog, there is recent evidence that an amacrine cell can be interposed between a rod bipolar cell and a ganglion cell, thus making the straight-through pathway a four-neuron chain. In the cat the rod bipolar cells seem to be connected to the ganglion cell via an amacrine cell, constituting a clear example of a four-neuron chain (Kolb and Famiglietti, 1974).

Lateral pathways

Lateral pathways exist in the photoreceptor layer, the outer plexiform layer and the inner plexiform layer

In the photoreceptor layer there are direct contacts between photoreceptor

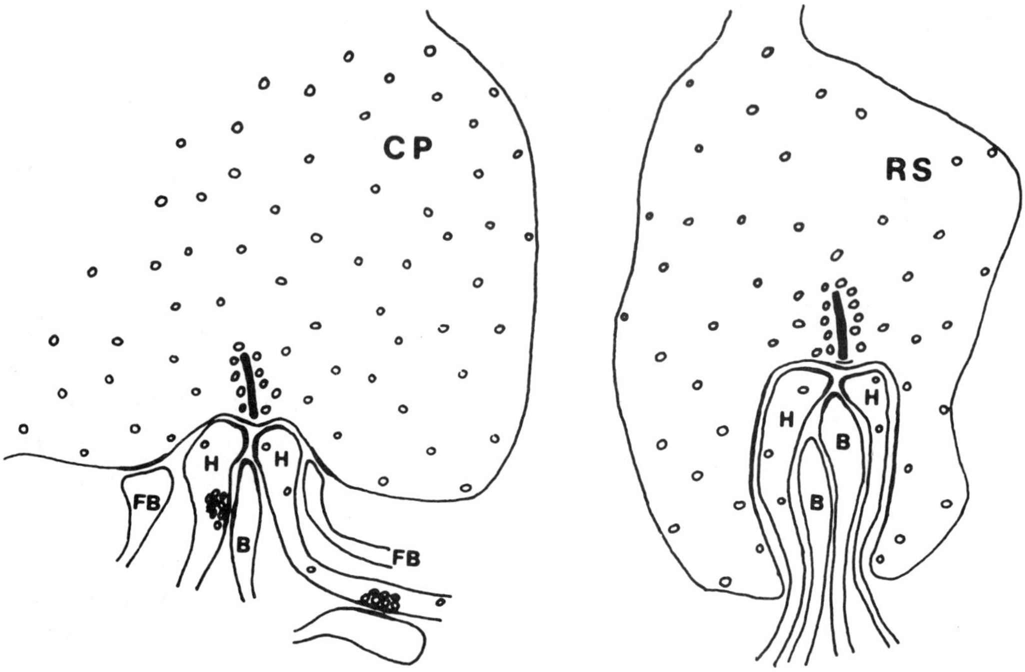

Fig. 1.3. Schematic presentation of rod and cone synapses. The rod spherule (RS), shown at the right, has in the invagination opposite the synaptic ribbon two horizontal cell processes (H) and two bipolar cell dendrites (B) as postsynaptic elements. The cone pedicle (CP), shown at the left, has numerous (up to 25) ribbon synapses, only one of which is shown. A triad of postsynaptic elements, consisting of two horizontal cell processes (H) and a central bipolar cell dendrite (B), is directly opposite the ribbon. In addition, two flat type bipolars (FB) are in "flat contact" with the pedicle.
After Dubin, 1973.

cells, both between rods and cones as well as between rods. The function of these direct contacts, which seem to be electrical synapses, is not yet clear (Stell, 1972). In the outer plexiform layer the horizontal cells interconnect different receptor cells. Two types of horizontal cells are known: those which have an axon and dendrite-like processes, and those which have dendrite-like processes only. The dendrite endings are in synaptic contact with cones only, and the axonal endings with rods only. There are also synaptic contacts between two horizontal cells.

In the inner plexiform layer the amacrine cells provide the lateral connections, e.g. between a bipolar and a ganglion cell. Amacrine cells never have an axon, but they have processes, which may be both presynaptic and postsynaptic elements within the inner plexiform layer: postsynaptic to bipolar cells, either post- or presynaptic to other amacrine cells, and presynaptic in synapses with bipolar and ganglion cells.

Synapses in the outer plexiform layer

Synapses involving receptor cells are either of the ribbon type or the flat contact type, both shown in Fig. 1.3. The ribbon synapse is characterized by a dense ribbon or bar in the presynaptic cytoplasm. The bar is surrounded by an array of synaptic vesicles and is oriented at right angles to the adjacent plasma membrane. There are always several (three to five) postsynaptic elements. The flat synapse has little synaptic specialization, no ribbon or cluster of synaptic vesicles, and is formed by two flat membrane surfaces opposing each other. A detailed study of the organization of the synapses by means of freeze-fracture electron-microscopy has recently been published by Raviola and Gilula (1975).

The conventional type of synapse, characterized by a group of vesicles near the presynaptic membrane, presynaptic and postsynaptic specialization and cleft specialization (Fig. 1.1), is found in the outer plexiform layer only where a horizontal cell process is the presynaptic element. In this case the postsynaptic element is either another horizontal cell process, a bipolar cell dendrite or, rarely, a bipolar cell body, but never a receptor cell. These conventional type synapses have never been found in the outer plexiform layer of human or monkey retina, rarely in that of lower mammals, frequently in that of amphibian retina. An exception is formed by the recently discovered interplexiform neuron, which in the Cebus monkey does form conventional synapses in both plexiform layers (Dowling and Ehinger, 1975).

Synapses in the inner plexiform layer

The types of synapses found in the inner plexiform layer are shown schematically in Fig. 1.2. The bipolar cells always have synaptic ribbons in their terminations, but the amacrine cells never have ribbon-type synaptic terminations. There are usually two postsynaptic elements (a dyad) at each bipolar cell synapse, one element containing vesicles and the other empty. The vesicle-containing element is an amacrine cell process, and the empty element is a ganglion cell dendrite. One sees also dyads consisting of two amacrine cells or two ganglion cells. Finally there are dyads, which are the presynaptic elements in a conventional synapse with a bipolar cell, the latter being called a "reciprocal synapse". There are also conventional synapses involving a series of three to five cells, where an amacrine cell is presynaptic to another amacrine cell, which is presynaptic to a ganglion cell dendrite, etc., a so-called "serial synapse". Finally, there is evidence in birds that there are efferent fibers entering the retina through the optic nerve, which form conventional synapses with amacrine and perhaps ganglion cells in the inner plexiform layer.

Quantitative studies for different species indicate that the lower species have more complex receptive fields with higher proportions of conventional (amacrine cell) synapses and of serial synapses than the higher species of vertebrates.

Central pathways of the visual system

The two central pathways of the visual system conduct the retinal impulses from the two eyes to the brain, which subject is discussed in considerable detail by Brindley (1970). The ganglion cell axons converge in the optic fiber layer to the *papilla*, where they leave the retina and the eye through the *optic nerve*. The optic nerves from the two eyes converge in the *optic chiasm*, where they cross and continue as the *optic tracts* to the *lateral geniculate nucleus*, the primary visual center. In the latter structure the fibers form synapses with another set of neurons, which carry the retinal impulses to the *visual cortex*. The retinal surfaces are projected two-dimensionally on the lateral geniculate nucleus and from there on the visual cortex. This is illustrated schematically in Fig. 1.4.

Part of each optic nerve branches off after the optic chiasm and carries a number of fibers to the *superior colliculus*, which serves as a center for light reflexes and for the correlation of impulses from the retina with movements of the skeletal muscles.

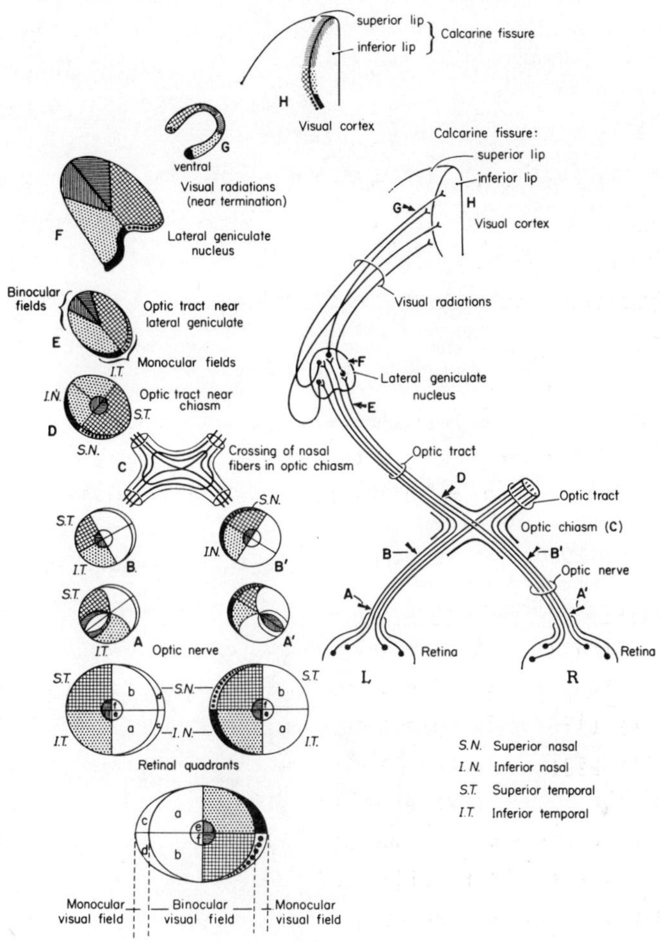

Fig. 1.4. The central pathway of the visual system with the optical projection of the retinal surfaces. After Crosby et al. (1962).

MECHANISM OF THE VERTEBRATE VISUAL SYSTEM

The process may be summarized in the following way. The retinal image formation involves three successive stages: the first image is formed in the photoreceptor cells, the second within the bipolars, and the final one within the ganglion cells. In the formation of the second image the horizontal cells alter the form of the signal, while the amacrine cells alter the form of the signal arriving in the ganglion cells. Thereafter the signal is conducted by the optic nerve and optic tract to the visual cortex. The present account must of necessity be brief and simplified, but a more detailed account is presented by Rodieck (1973) and Werblin (1973).

Photoreceptor cells

The structure of a vertebrate rod is shown schematically in Fig. 1.5. Its two main parts are the outer and the inner segments. The outer segment contains a stack of some 500-2000 flat rod sacs, while the inner segment contains

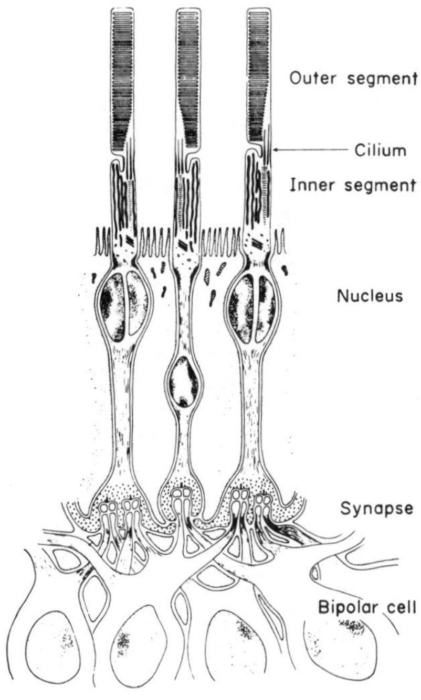

Fig. 1.5. Structure of vertebrate rod photoreceptor cell

mitochondria, endoplasmic reticulum, nucleus and ends in the rod spherule with its synaptic contacts. The outer and inner segment are connected by the narrow cilium. The rod sacs, which are not connected with the outer segment outer membrane, contain the visual pigment rhodopsin. The major difference between a cone and a rod is that in the cone the sacs are replaced by numerous deep invaginations of the outer membrane.

Our knowledge of the biochemical events in the photoreceptor cell upon illumination is most extensive for the rod, since they can be easily isolated in bulk. For comprehensive reviews two volumes of the Handbook of Sensory Physiology (Dartnall, 1972; Fuortes, 1972) should be consulted, while two shorter reviews by the present author (Bonting, 1969; Bonting, 1974) may be mentioned. The main events can be briefly summarized as follows.

The rod sac membrane or photoreceptor membrane consists of a lipid bilayer of high fluidity, in which the rhodopsin molecules diffuse and rotate freely. Rhodopsin is a protein of M.W. 39,000 with 11-cis retinaldehyde as a chromophoric group. It is the major protein component of the photoreceptor membrane, representing nearly 90% of total membrane protein. Its absorption spectrum is characterized by a peak at 500 nm with very high molar extinction, which upon illumination disappears and is replaced by one at 380 nm. During this change, which lasts only about a millisecond at 37°C, the chromophoric group isomerizes to the all-trans configuration and the molecule is converted via three very short-lived intermediates (prelumirhodopsin , lumirhodopsin, and metarhodopsin I) into metarhodopsin II (λ_{max} = 380 nm), which is stable for several minutes.

The conversion of rhodopsin to metarhodopsin II leads to a crucial, though as yet undetermined change in the photoreceptor membrane. This change affects the outer membrane of the outer segment, from which it is separated by a gap of at least 70 Å, hence it seems likely that a transmitter substance is involved (see chapter 3). There is a very drastic reduction in the sodium permeability of the latter membrane. In darkness an electric current is running along the rod photoreceptor from the inner to the outer segment; it is carried by sodium ions, which are actively extruded by a sodium pump in the inner segment membrane and passively admitted through the outer segment membrane. The decrease in sodium permeability of this membrane leads to a decrease in the dark current and a hyperpolarization of the membrane, which spreads to the synapse and activates it.

All vertebrate photoreceptors, rods as well as cones, hyperpolarize upon illumination. The response is a graded one over a 3000-fold intensity range, above which it saturates. In rods a response is first detected at a flux of about 5 photons per cell per second, while in cones of the order of 100 photons per cell per second are required. The rod response does not turn off when the test flash ends, but it returns only slowly to the dark level. Measurable bleaching of the photopigment requires light intensities about 10^7x higher than threshold intensity. The response range for cones is shifted by background illumination; hence they generate good responses to changes in intensity around the background level, but the absolute level of the background is not well represented. The rod response curves do not shift, so at low intensities below saturation rods represent absolute background levels better.

Bipolar cells

The photoreceptor cells drive the bipolar and horizontal cells. The bipolar cells appear to be passively awaiting the results of synaptic interactions between receptors and horizontal cells. In the foveal area the bipolars contact only one photoreceptor with their dendritic processes, while in the periphery a single bipolar may contact many photoreceptors.

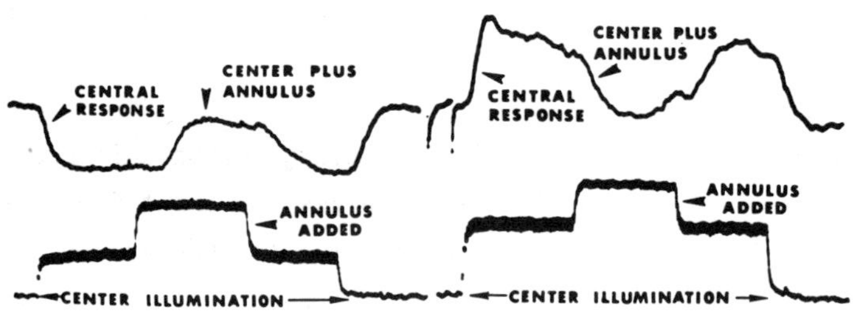

Fig. 1.6. Bipolar cell responses: hyperpolarizing and depolarizing type. The cells are polarized first by a test flash at the center. Then, in the presence of the test flash, an annulus is added. This largely abolishes the center response in either type. Finally, the annulus is terminated, whereupon the central response returns. After Werblin and Dowling (1969).

The bipolar cells are driven through two pathways. A small spot of light centered on the photoreceptor will activate the receptor-bipolar pathway. A ring surrounding a certain bipolar cell will illuminate receptors that drive horizontal cells in contact with this bipolar.

The electrical response of the bipolar cell is always a graded, slow-potential response. Two types of bipolar cells can be distinguished: one that depolarizes upon steady central illumination, and one that hyperpolarizes (Fig. 1.6.). Addition of an annulus reduces the response to central illumination in both cases.

The decrease in the bipolar response upon surround illumination may be due to a depolarizing effect of a hyperpolarized horizontal cell on a nearby photoreceptor cell, which may represent a feedback pathway from horizontal to photoreceptor cell modulating the receptor signal.

Ganglion cells

The electrical responses of a ganglion cell consists of a series of spikes, typical for neurons which must transmit signals over long distances. Here again two different types of cells may be distinguished on the basis of the electrical response: a tonic or "on" type and a phasic or "off" type (Fig. 1.7). The first type gives a sustained slow potential and steady discharge of spikes upon central illumination. Surround illumination drives the membrane potential back toward the resting level and inhibits firing. The second type gives transient responses both at the onset and the cessation of illumination.

The similarity between the responses of the tonic ganglion cell and of the bipolar cell suggests that the tonic cell receives its input from one or very few bipolar cells only. The phasic cell would seem to receive its main input from an amacrine cell, which always depolarizes upon stimulation. Both types of ganglion cells show, initially at least, a depolarizing response.

The tonic or "on" ganglion cell, like the bipolar cell, seems to indicate the relative level of illumination in the center of its receptive field, and its sensitivity is controlled by the average steady illumination levels in surrounding regions. The sensitivity of the phasic of "off" ganglion cell, on the other hand, is altered by interactions at both plexiform layers. It may act as a spatial contrast detector or as a temporal change detector.

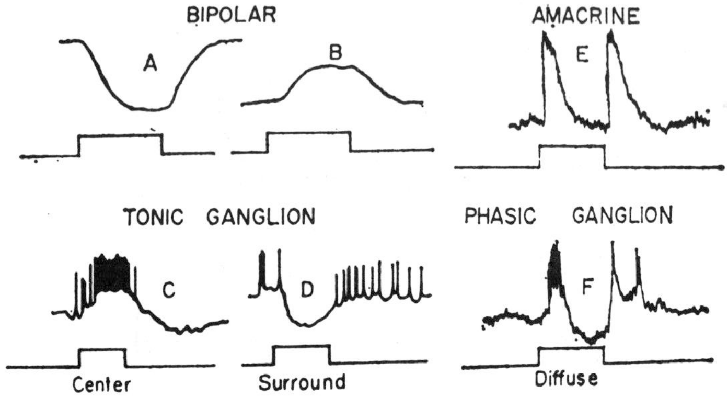

Fig. 1.7. Ganglion cell responses, compared with those of bipolar and amacrine cells. The tonic ganglion cell response to central (C) and annular (D) stimulation appears to reflect that of the bipolar cell (A and B). The phasic ganglion cell response (F) reflects that of the amacrine cell (E).
After Werblin (1973).

Correlation of electrical responses and synaptic organization

The synaptic organization of the retina can now be correlated with the electrical responses of the various cells described before (Dowling, 1970). The lefthand receptor in Fig. 1.8 is thought to receive a flash of light, the righthand receptor a continuous, dim background illumination. The rod receptor cells behave relatively autonomously in the sense that they respond very slightly to light falling on surrounding receptor cells, and this small response is probably due to stray light. For cones there is evidence for feedback from horizontal cells in the turtle (Baylor et al., 1971).

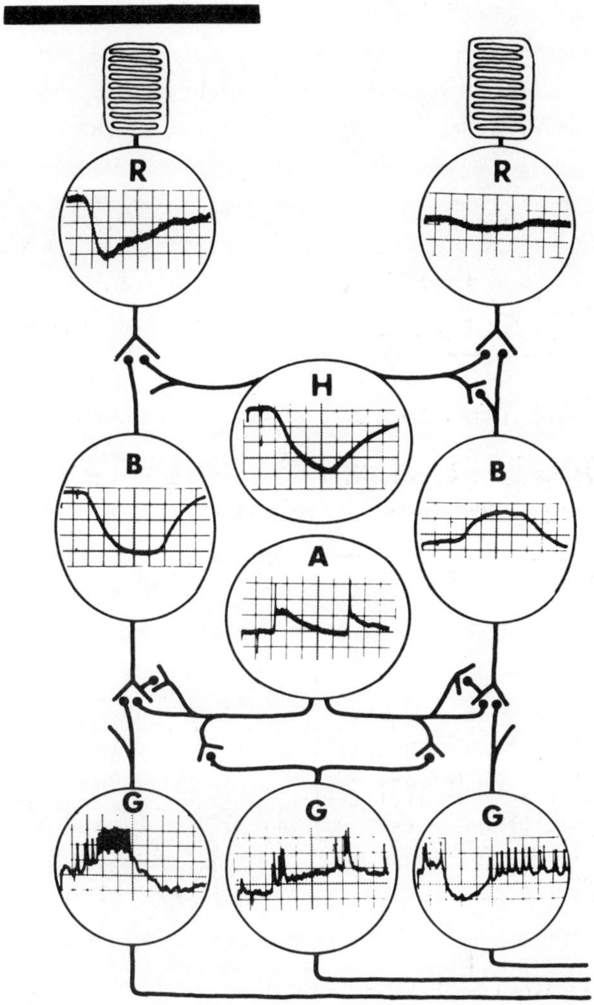

Fig. 1.8. Correlation of synaptic organization of the vertebrate retina with intracellularly recorded responses of the neurons. R, photoreceptor cell; H, horizontal cell; B, bipolar cell; A, amacrine cell; G, ganglion cell. The left receptor is receiving a light flash, while the right receptor is exposed to a steady, low-intensity background illumination.
After Dowling (1970).

Horizontal cells integrate the input from a wide area. The latencies of horizontal cell and bipolar cell responses match closely, indicating that both are driven by the receptors. Bipolar dendrites and horizontal cell processes are activated together at the synaptic ribbon synapses of the receptors.

Bipolar cells are polarized strongly in a graded, sustained fashion by direct contacts with receptors. This polarization is antagonized by horizontal cells, acting on bipolar cell dendrites (Fig. 1.8, right). This interaction may occur at the horizontal-bipolar synapses, but also in the receptor synapses.

The central response in bipolar cells is mediated by direct receptor-bipolar contacts; the antagonistic surround response by horizontal-bipolar contacts. The amacrine cells do not appear to be involved, since they respond transiently to both on and off illumination, while the surround inhibition in the bipolar cell response is graded and sustained, similar to the form of the horizontal cell response.

The transient response of the amacrine cells to the sustained responses of the bipolar cells may be due to their special synaptic relationship. The reciprocal synapses of the amacrine cell processes back onto the bipolar terminals, just adjacent to the bipolar ribbon synapses to the ganglion cells, may turn off the bipolar excitation locally, resulting in a transient response in the amacrine cell.

The two types of ganglion cell responses, "on" and "off" type, may be related to the character of the input into each kind of cell. The "on" type has a receptive field organization similar to that of the bipolar cells (left and right ganglion cells in Fig. 1.8). Central illumination causes sustained depolarization of the cell, while surround illumination inhibits the activity in a sustained fashion. This cell receives most of its synaptic input directly from the bipolar terminals.

The "off" type of ganglion cell (center ganglion cell in Fig. 1.8) responds transiently to retinal illumination, like the amacrine cells, and presumably receives its major synaptic input from the amacrine cells. This is the complex that seems to function in detecting motion. The outer plexiform layer appears concerned mainly with the static or spatial aspects of the illumination on the receptors, while the inner plexiform layer is concerned more with the dynamic or temporal aspects. Amacrine cells respond vigorously to moving stimuli. The two types of ganglion cells appear to be closely related to either the bipolar or amacrine cell activity, and to carry the information on the transformations occurring at the two plexiform layers to the higher visual centers.

It should be emphasized that our understanding of the functioning of the retinal network is by no means complete at this time. Hence, the account given here may still have to be amended on various points in the next few years.

Central pathway

Most of the trains of spikes generated in the ganglion cells by the photons absorbed in the photoreceptors travel through the million or so nerve fibers of the optic nerve to the lateral geniculate nucleus, from which they are relayed to the visual cortex. A smaller number travels to the superior colliculus, which is involved in visually guided movements. The responses obtained from single geniculate cells after light stimulation of the retina are remarkably similar to those obtained from the ganglion cells. This means that there is little or no recoding or discarding of any information present in the discharges of optic nerve fibers. The transmitters involved at the late lateral geniculate nucleus and the superior colliculus are discussed in Chapter 9.

CONCLUDING REMARKS

Even from this simplified account of the structure and mechanism of the visual system it will be obvious that the investigator, who wants to determine which transmitter is involved at each point where a signal has to cross the gap between two adjacent excitable membranes, faces a tremendous task but also a great challenge! There are 7 types of cells, which are connected in many different ways by 3 types of synapses, at which in principle about any of a dozen different substances could act as the transmitter. The next nine chapters will report the remarkable progress that has been made to date, but also the many questions, uncertainties and problems still facing us. The contributors to this symposium volume hope that many who read it will be stimulated to join the effort.

REFERENCES

Bachelard H.S. (1974) Brain Biochemistry, Chapman and Hall, London

Baylor D.A., Fuortes M.G.F. and O'Bryan P.M. (1971) Receptive fields of cones in the retina of the turtle. J. Physiol. 214, 265-294

Bonting S.L. (1969) The mechanism of the visual process. Curr. Topics in Bioenergetics 3, 351-415

Bonting S.L. (1974) Biochemistry of visual pigments in relation to visual excitation, in Biochemistry of Sensory Functions (Jaenicke L., ed.), pp. 1-21. Springer-Verlag, Berlin

Brindley G.S. (1970) Physiology of the Retina and Visual Pathway. Second ed., pp. 90-131. Arnold Publishers, London

Brown G.L., Dale H.H. and Feldberg W. (1936) Reactions of the normal mammalian muscle to acetylcholine and eserine. J. Physiol. 87, 394-424

Cajal S.R. (1972) The Structure of the Retina (Thorpe S.A. and Glickstein M., trans.) Thomas, Springfield, Ill.

Crosby E.C., Humphrey T. and Lauer E.W. (1962) Correlative Anatomy of the Nervous System. Macmillan, New York

Curtis D.R. (1964) Microelectrophoresis, in Physical Techniques in Biological Research (Nastuk W.L., ed.) Vol. 5A, pp. 144-190. Acad. Press, New York

Curtis D.R. and Johnston G.A.R. (1973) Amino acid transmitters in the mammalian nervous system. Ergebn. der Physiologie 69, 98-188

Dale H.H. (1935) Pharmacology and nerve-endings. Proc. Roy. Soc. Med. Med. 28, 319-332

Dale H.H., Feldberg W. and Vogt M. (1936) Release of acetylcholine at voluntary motor nerve endings. J. Physiol. 86, 353-380

Dartnall H.J.A. (1972) Handbook of Sensory Physiology: Photochemistry of Vision, Vol. VII/1. Springer-Verlag, Berlin

De Robertis E., de Iraldi A.P., de Lores Arnaiz G.R. and Salganicof L. (1962) Cholinergic and non-cholinergic nerve endings in rat brain. J. Neurochem. 9, 23-35

Dowling J.E. (1970) Organization of vertebrate retinas. Invest. Ophth. 9, 655-680

Dowling J.E. and Ehinger B. (1975) Synaptic organization of the amine-containing interplexiform cells of the goldfish and Cebus monkey retinas. Science 188, 270-273

Dubin M.W. (1974) Anatomy of the vertebrate retina, in The Eye (Davson H. and Graham Jr. L.T., eds.) Vol. 6, pp. 227-256. Acad. Press, New York

Falck B. (1962) Observations on the possibility of the cellular localisation of monoamines by a fluorescent method. Acta Physiol. Scand. 56, suppl. 197

Fuchs F. (1974) Striated muscle. Ann. Rev. Physiol. 36, 461-502

Fuortes M.G.F. (1972) Handbook of Sensory Physiology: Physiology of Photoreceptor Organs, Vol. VII/2. Springer-Verlag, Berlin

Goldberg N.O., O'Dea R.F. and Haddox M.K. (1973) Cyclic GMP, in Advances in Cyclic Nucleotide Research (Greengard P. and Robison G.A., eds.) Vol. 3, pp. 155-223. Raven Press, New York

Graham Jr. L.T. (1974) Comparative aspects of neurotransmitters in the retina, in The Eye (Davson H. and Graham Jr. L.T., eds.) Vol. 6, pp. 283-342. Acad. Press, New York

Gray E.G. and Whittaker V.P. (1962) The isolation of nerve endings from brain. J. Anat. Lond. 96, 79-88

Greengard P. and Kebabian J.W. (1974) Role of cyclic AMP in synaptic transmission in the mammalian peripheral nervous system. Federation Proc. 33, 1059-1067

Kolb H. and Famiglietti E.V. (1974) Rod and cone pathways in the inner plexiform layer of cat retina. Science 186, 47-49

Lajtha A. (1969-73) Handbook of Neurochemistry, Vols. 1-8, Plenum Press, New York

Langhan T.A. (1973) Protein kinases and protein kinase substrates, in Advances in Cyclic Nucleotide Research (Greengard P. and Robison G.A., eds.) Vol. 3, pp. 99-154. Raven Press, New York

Marchbanks R.M. and Whittaker V.P. (1969) The biochemistry of synaptosomes, in Biological Basis of Medicine (Bittar E.E. and Bittar N., eds.) Vol. 1, pp. 39-76. Acad. Press, New York

Raviola E. and Gilula N.B. (1975) Intramembrane organization of specialized contacts in the outer plexiform layer of the retina. A freeze-fracture study in monkeys and rabbits. J. Cell Biol. 65, 192-222

Robison G.A., Butcher R.W. and Sutherland E.W. (1971) Cyclic AMP. Acad. Press, New York

Rodieck R.W. (1973) The Vertebrate Retina, Principles of Structure and Function. Freeman, San Francisco

Schultz G., Hardman J.G., Schultz K., Baird C.E. and Sutherland C.W. (1973) The importance of calcium ions for the regulation of guanisine 3'5' cyclic monophosphate levels. Proc. Nat. Acad. Sci. USA 70, 3889-3893

Stell W.K. (1972) The morphological organization of the vertebrate retina, in Handbook of Sensory Physiology: Physiology of Photoreceptor Organs (Fuortes M.G.F., ed.) Vol. VII/2, pp. 112-213. Springer-Verlag, Berlin

Thorn N.A. and Petersen O.H. (1974) Secretory Mechanisms of Exocrine Glands, pp. 305-407. Munksgaard, Copenhagen; Acad. Press, New York

Werblin F.S. (1973) Organization of the vertebrate retina, in The Eye (Davson H. and Graham Jr. L.T., eds.) Vol. 6, pp. 257-281. Acad. Press, New York

Werblin F.S. and Dowling J.E. (1969) Organization of the retina of the mudpuppy, Necturus maculosus. II. Intra-recordings J. Neurophysiol. 32, 339-355

White A., Handler Ph. and Smith E.L. (1973) Principles of Biochemistry, 5th ed., McGraw-Hill, New York

CHAPTER 2

ROLE OF CYCLIC NUCLEOTIDES IN PHOTORECEPTOR FUNCTION

C. Goridis, N. Virmaux, M. Weller and P.F. Urban

Centre de Neurochimie, CNRS
67085 Strasbourg Cédex, France

Present addresses:
Dr. C. Goridis: CNRS - CBM4, 13274 Marseille Cédex 2, France
Dr. M. Weller: Dept. of Chemical Pathology, Univ. of Stellenbosch, Tygerberg Hospital, Parowvallei 7503, Cape Town, South Africa

INTRODUCTION

The function of the rod outer segment, the photosensitive part of the rod photoreceptor cell, comprises two different tasks : the detection of photons and the translation of photon capture into a signal which can be transported and processed by nerve cells. The latter process involves membrane conductivity changes. Whereas great progress has been made in elucidating the photochemical reactions occurring in rod outer segments (see Bonting, this book, ch. 1), very little is known as to how photon capture and the subsequent bleaching reactions of the rhodopsin molecule are able to induce a neuronal signal in the photoreceptor cell. The first detectable event following photonic stimulation is a transient change of the sodium conductance of the rod membrane envelope. In vertebrate rod outer segments, the dark state is accompanied by a constant inward current of Na^+ into the organelle and this dark current is decreased as a result of illumination (Sillman et al., 1969b ; Yoshikami and Hagins, 1973). But photoreceptor function calls not only for a process which links chromophore bleaching to changes of the Na^+-entry, but also for a system which enables the outer segments to detect photons against a background of widely differing light intensities, i.e. a mechanism which modulates photoreceptor sensitivity.

There are a number of reasons why cyclic nucleotides could be suspected of being involved in either the transduction of photon capture into changes of outer segment permeability, or in the modulation of photoreceptor sensitivity. (1) In vertebrate rod outer segments, rhodopsin bleaching and changes in Na^+-conductance occur on anatomically distinct sites : most of the rhodopsin is contained in the membrane of closed, flattened sacs (or discs), which are separated from the plasma membrane by a space of at least 100 nm (Cohen, 1970 ; Hagins, 1972). Hence, control of rod outer membrane conductivity by rhodopsin bleaching calls for a second messenger because of the structural separation of the two events. (2) In visual excitation, an enormous amplification is needed since a single absorbed photon can transiently reduce a rod's dark current by about 3 percent (Cone and Pak, 1971) ; the cyclic AMP system is a most impressive example of a biological amplification device.

Table 2.1. Guanylate cyclase activity in various tissues and structures

	Enzyme activity[(a)]	
Rat brain[(b)]	31 ± 3.3	(5)
Rat brain synaptoplasm[(b)]	239 ± 58	(5)
Rat liver	12 ± 0.7	(11)
Rat liver plasma membranes[(c)]	12 ± 0.8	(8)
Rabbit kidney cortex[(d)]	29 ± 2.3	(8)
Rabbit kidney glomeruli[(d)]	414 ± 40	(8)
Bovine brain	25 ± 1.2	(4)
Bovine retina	170 ± 2.8	(8)
Bovine retina soluble fraction[(e)]	132 ± 1.4	(6)
Bovine retina particulate fraction[(e)]	286 ± 8.4	(6)
Bovine rod outer segments	2,652 ±165	(7)

(a) Expressed as pmole cyclic GMP formed/min/mg protein with S.E. and nr. of expts.;
(b) From Goridis and Morgan (1973);
(c) From Goridis and Reutter (1975);
(d) From Helwig et al. (1975);
(e) From Goridis et al. (1973).

(3) Cyclic AMP appears to regulate sodium permeability of the plasma membrane in toad bladder (De Lorenzo et al., 1973) and there is rather compelling evidence that cyclic AMP and cyclic GMP are modulating neuronal excitability in a number of systems such as cerebellar Purkinje cells (Hoffer et al., 1972), cerebral cortex (Stone et al., 1975) and the superior cervical ganglion (Greengard et al., 1972).

If cyclic nucleotides are to play a role in either the transduction of photon capture into changes of plasma membrane permeability or in the modulation of photoreceptor sensitivity, the enzymes responsible for their formation (adenylate cyclase or guanylate cyclase) and degradation (cyclic nucleotide phosphodiesterases) should be associated with the photoreceptors. Indeed, our very first experiments (Table 2.1) showed that highly purified bovine rod outer segments contain a guanylate cyclase with a specific activity higher than any previously recorded in any tissue preparation by us (Goridis et al., 1973; Goridis and Morgan, 1973) or by other authors (White and Aurbach, 1969; Hardman and Sutherland, 1969; Kimura and Murad, 1975). A high cyclic GMP phosphodiesterase activity has also been found in purified outer segments (Pannbacker et al., 1972; Goridis and Virmaux, 1974; Chader et al., 1974a). By contrast, retinal adenylate cyclase does not appear to be enriched in photoreceptor organelles although low activities might still be associated with the rods (Hendriks et al., 1973; Manthorpe and McConnell, 1974). Originally, light-sensitivity of this enzyme has been reported (Bitensky et al., 1971; Miller et al., 1971). This effect has now been recognized as caused by inadequate control of cyclic nucleotide degradation in the assay system (Miki et al., 1973; Miki et al., 1974). Therefore, cyclic GMP rather than cyclic AMP appears to be the cyclic nucleotide implicated in rod function.

Among the many questions raised by the presence of high cyclic GMP synthetizing and hydrolyzing activities in rod outer segments, the present report attempts to answer the following ones. (1) Is the extremely active guanylate cyclase intrinsic to the outer segments ? (2) Are the enzyme activities involved in cyclic GMP metabolism light-sensitive ? (3) Is the protein kinase activity of rod outer segments controlled by cyclic nucleotides ? (4) Is the endogenous cyclic GMP content of the rod cells influenced by low, physiological levels of bleaching ? If so, is the time course of the observed changes compatible with a role of cyclic GMP in visual excitation ?

METHODOLOGY

The major disadvantage in working with photosensitive material is the requirement to exclude photochemical reactions prior to or during experiment. Therefore, all operations, except intentional illuminations, were carried out in dim red light. Only buffer extracts of photoreceptor material and preparations derived from them, which do not contain rhodopsin, were handled in the light. Cattle eyes were excised within 10 min of slaughter and stored on ice in a light-tight box for 2 hr. Frog retinae were obtained from *Ranae esculentae*, which had been dark-adapted overnight.

Highly purified rod outer segments were prepared as previously described (Virmaux et al., 1971). The purity of the rod outer segments was characterized by the spectral ratio A_{280} : A_{500}, the ratios obtained (2.2 - 2.3) indicate excellent purity (Hendriks et al., 1973; Hemminki, 1974). Incubation with 11-*cis*-retinaldehyde only increased the optical density at 500 nm by 5-10 percent, indicating that the material was maximally 10 percent bleached. If the distribution of guanylate cyclase in various retina fractions was to be determined, the 67 mM phosphate buffer used during preparation of the outer segments was replaced by 100 mM Tris-acetic acid (pH 7.4), since phosphate at this concentration inhibits guanylate cyclase. Centrifugation of purified outer segments on continuous sucrose gradients was performed as previously described (Virmaux et al., 1975).

Rhodopsin was purified by sequential extraction of the rod outer segments with 10 mM Tris-HCl buffer and low concentrations of sodium dodecylsulfate (Weller et al., 1975). The insoluble material was washed exhaustively to remove the detergent. The rhodopsin preparation thus obtained, though not representing pure rhodopsin, contains no protein other than opsin as judged by polyacrylamide gel electrophoresis (Virmaux et al., 1972). The initial buffer wash of the rod preparation served as a convenient source of cyclic nucleotide phosphodiesterase and protein kinase. Cyclic nucleotide phosphodiesterase was purified from these buffer extracts by successive chromatography on DEAE-cellulose and Sephadex G100 (Coquil et al., 1975). This simple purification scheme removed more than 97 percent of the protein present in the hypotonic extract. The resulting enzyme preparations showed a high, but variable specific activity towards cyclic GMP (1.1 - 7.0 μmole GMP formed/min/mg protein with 10 μM cyclic GMP as substrate).

For determination of the endogenous cyclic nucleotide content, intact frog or cattle retinae were incubated *in vitro*. Calf retinae were incubated in a glucose-containing bicarbonate-buffered medium, pre-equilibrated with 5% CO_2 - 95% O_2. The retinae were incubated at 37°C with continuous gassing with the same gas mixture. At the end of a 60 min preincubation, the retinae were placed individually into 10 ml Erlenmeyer flasks containing 3.5 ml fresh medium. After 12 min, the retinae were rapidly removed and dropped into 3.5 ml 1M $HClO_4$. This operation was done in less than 5 sec. After homogenisation and centrifugation to remove the protein precipitate, the extracts were neutralized with K_2CO_3 and stored at -20°C until determination of the cyclic GMP content.

Frog retinae were superfused at room temperature with oxygenated (95% O_2 - 5% CO_2) frog Ringer-solution containing 80 mM NaCl, 2 mM KCl, 0.1 mM $CaCl_2$, 0.1 mM $MgCl_2$, 15 mM sodium phosphate buffer (pH 7.8), and 5 mM glucose (3.5 ml/min). Two different conditions were used : (1) the retinae were superfused in a small cylindrical glass chamber and illuminated by a non-attenuated flash-light (maximum energy 15 J, duration 1 msec, distance 1.5 cm), which gave essentially full bleaching; (2) the retinae were mounted in a perfusion chamber and illuminated by an attenuated flash-light (maximum energy 27 J, attenuated to log-3.0 by a neutral density filter, duration 1 msec, distance 2 cm). In both cases, the flash was given after a preliminary 30 min period of superfusion and the reaction stopped at various times thereafter by rapid injection of 0.33 M $HClO_4$. Dark-values are obtained by stopping the reaction at 30 min. They remained essentially constant between 20 and 50 min of superfusion. The earliest time points are determined by the time necessary for injection of the acid and its arrival in the chamber. Considering the location of the rods at the surface of the retina, the time necessary for diffusion into the rods should be negligible. Difference spectra before and after exhaustive bleaching were recorded on crude homogenates of retinae superfused and illuminated under the same conditions (Frank et al., 1973).

The cyclic GMP in neutralized retina extracts was estimated by radioimmunoassay, using a slight modification (Goridis et al., 1974) of the method of Cailla et al. (1975). In some cases, cyclic AMP was determined on the same extracts by an analogous technique (Cailla et al., 1973).

Guanylate cyclase activity was measured with 0.185 mM $\alpha[^{32}P]$GTP as substrate in the presence of optimum concentrations of Mn^{++} as previously described (Helwig et al., 1975). The reaction mixture contained unlabeled cyclic GMP (7mM) to minimize degradation of cyclic $[^{32}P]$GMP by phosphodiesterase and the extent of the degradation was checked routinely by addition of cyclic $[^{3}H]$GMP. All values, where measurable hydrolysis of cyclic GMP during the incubation period had occurred, were discarded. In later experiments, the phosphodiesterase inhibitor SQ 20,009 (kindly supplied by Dr S.M. Hess, Squibb Institute of Medical Research) was added (0.35 mM). In the presence of this effective inhibitor of cyclic GMP hydrolysis (see Table 2.10) unlabeled cyclic GMP still had to be included in the incubation mixture to prevent degradation of the [^{32}P] cyclic GMP formed. When low activities were to be measured, the eluate from the Al_2O_3 column was further chromatographed on Dowex 1X2 (formate form). This step is very effective in lowering the blank values to levels below 0.006 percent of total [^{32}P] counts.

Phosphodiesterase activity was determined by the method of Thompson and Appleman (1971) with 1 mM cyclic nucleotide as substrate or by the method of Schultz et al. (1974) in the case of lower substrate concentrations. Incubations were performed at 30°C for 4 min. For each enzyme preparation different dilutions were tested to assure that the reaction velocity was proportional to enzyme concentrations. All values, where more than 20 percent of the substrate had been metabolized, were discarded. Enzyme assays were carried out at least in duplicate and results are given as average values.

Phosphorylation of rod outer segment protein was measured as described by Weller et al. (1975). The ATP concentration was 1 mM. For estimation of protein phosphatase activity intact outer segments were phosphorylated by incubation with [^{32}P] ATP, washed free of non-covalently bound radioactivity and incubated in 50 mM Tris-HCl (pH 7.4).

GUANYLATE CYCLASE OF ROD OUTER SEGMENTS

Following our initial discovery of an extremely rapid rate of cyclic GMP formation in isolated outer segments (Table 2.1), we designed experiments to prove that this high activity was indeed associated with the photoreceptor organelles. To this aim, we measured guanylate cyclase activity and rhodopsin content associated with various fractions derived from retinal homogenates during isolation of the outer segments. The method used for purification of these organelles is aimed at obtaining the highest possible purity and losses of rod material during the fractionation procedure are therefore unavoidable. Using the recovery of rhodopsin (only minor quantities of rhodopsin occur outside the outer segments) as reference, allowance

Table 2.2 Distribution of guanylate cyclase activity and unbleached rhodopsin in retinal fractions

Fraction	Guanylate cyclase		Rhodopsin	
	enrichment	Percent of total activity	enrichment	Percent of total content
Retinal homogenate	1	100	1	100
2000 x g supernatant	2.42	88	2.07	76
25 000 x g supernatant	0.82	22	0.45	12
25 000 x g pellet	6.40	60	6.39	60
1st gradient, outer segments	12.5	47	13.0	51
1st gradient, top and middle	1.61	2.7	n.d.	
1st gradient, pellet	0.47	1.4	n.d.	
2nd gradient, outer segments	15.7	38	17.2	42

n.d. = not determined. Concentrations of unbleached rhodopsin were determined according to Manthorpe and Mc Connell (1974) except that 1.5 percent Emulphogene was used as detergent.

can be made for these losses. The guanylate cyclase activity of calf retina was remarkably concentrated in purified photoreceptors and the enrichment in the various fractions during isolation of outer segments was parallel to the rise in rhodopsin content. As shown in Table 2.2, 38 percent of the guanylate cyclase activity originally present in the retinal homogenate and 42 percent of the rhodopsin were recovered with the purest fraction, indicating that 90 percent of retinal guanylate cyclase is associated with the outer segments. A discrepancy between enzyme activity and rhodopsin content was seen only in the 25,000 x g supernatant, which contains relatively more guanylate cyclase. Allowance being made for the presence of rod outer segment fragments in this fraction, the activity which could be contributed by inner retinal structures represents only 10 percent of the total retinal activity. To strengthen the evidence that the activity measured in the highly purified outer segments was native to these organelles, the purest fraction was subjected to continuous gradient centrifugation. The peak of guanylate cyclase activity coincided with the peak of rhodopsin content and all guanylate cyclase activity sedimented with the rhodopsin bearing membranes (Fig. 2.1). The enzyme appeared to be firmly bound to the disc membranes, since it could not be washed off by low or high ionic strength buffers in combination with repeated freezing and thawing. Thus, in contrast to adenylate cyclase (Manthorpe and McConnell, 1974; Bownds et al. 1974), the high cyclic GMP forming capacity appears to be intrinsic to the disc membranes.

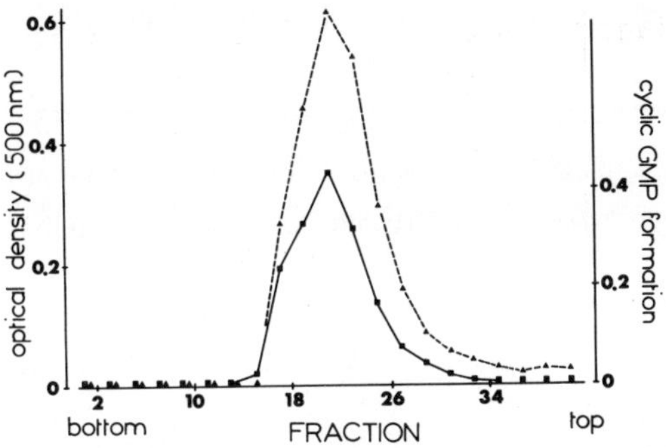

Fig. 2.1. Distribution of guanylate cyclase activity and rhodopsin in the fractions recovered by centrifugation of purified rod outer segments on a continuous sucrose gradient (16-37 percent sucrose). Rhodopsin content was estimated in the presence of 1.5 percent emulphogene by measuring the absorbancy at 500 nm (- - -). Guanylate cyclase activity is expressed as nmole cyclic GMP formed/min/fraction (——).

In our hands, this guanylate cyclase activity proved to be insensitive to light. In earlier experiments, outer segments which had been washed and taken up in hypotonic buffer, were used to eliminate partially the highly active cyclic GMP phosphodiesterase activity (Goridis et al., 1973). Hypotonic conditions, however, could have destroyed the structural integrity of the rods, which might be required to preserve light-sensitivity. In subsequent studies, addition of the phosphodiesterase inhibitor SQ 20,009 sufficiently prevented breakdown of the newly formed cyclic GMP to be able to repeat these experiments under isotonic conditions. Since regulatory properties of guanylate cyclase could have been lost during the lengthy purification procedure, a simplified method was adapted (Akhtar et al., 1968) allowing the testing for a possible light-effect within 3 hours after dissection of the retinae. Using outer segments purified in this manner, and even using a crude homogenate of calf retina, no effect of light-exposure on guanylate cyclase activity was found. In addition, cyclic GMP formation was estimated in intact retinae after prelabeling the nucleotide pool with [^{3}H]hypoxanthine. In the presence of the phosphodiesterase inhibitor SQ 20,009, easily measurable levels of [^{3}H]cyclic GMP accumulated, but no effect of light was observed (Goridis and Virmaux, 1974). Two accounts have been published, which confirm the presence of extremely high guanylate cyclase activities in rod outer segments, but which report light-inhibition of this enzyme (Pannbacker, 1973; Bensinger et al., 1974). Our attempts to reproduce these results have, however, been unsuccessful. In any case, the inhibition of cyclic GMP formation reported by Pannbacker (1973) occurs too slowly to account for the rapid changes of endogenous cyclic GMP levels observed in whole retina (see below).

LIGHT-REGULATED CYCLIC NUCLEOTIDE PHOSPHODIESTERASE IN BOVINE RETINA

Because of our failure to detect light-dependent changes of retinal cyclic GMP formation, we attempted to demonstrate an effect of light on cyclic GMP hydrolysis. Our initial experiments showed that cyclic GMP phosphodiesterase activity of retinal homogenates incubated in the light was more than three

Table 2.3 Effect of light on cyclic nucleotide phosphodiesterase in retina

	nmole 5' GMP formed/min/mg protein	
Preparation	light	dark
Bovine retina homogenate	29.0 ± 1.6 (9)	8.5 ± 0.8 (9)
Bovine rod outer segments	157	154
Rat brain homogenate	28.3	26.7
	nmole 5' AMP formed/mg protein/min	
	light	dark
Bovine retina homogenate	9.3 ± 0.6 (4)	6.3 ± 0.8 (4)

Retina homogenates (0.6 - 0.8 mg protein/assay) or suspensions of rod outer segments (50 µg protein/assay) were assayed for cyclic GMP phosphodiesterase activity in diffuse room light or complete darkness. Cyclic GMP or cyclic AMP (1 mM) were used as substrate. From Goridis and Virmaux (1974).

times that of homogenates assayed in the dark (Table 2.3). In later experiments, retina homogenates were exposed to light (5 min at $0^{o}C$, 33 W tungsten lamp, distance 4 cm) prior to the enzymatic assay which was carried out in dim red light. In these experiments, essentially the same activation was observed. As shown in Table 2.3, cyclic nucleotide phosphodiesterase of purified outer segments was not light-sensitive. As expected, illumination was without effect on brain phosphodiesterase. With cyclic AMP as substrate, a much smaller light-activation was seen.

Table 2.4. Effect of purified rhodopsin on retinal cyclic GMP phosphodiesterase

Preparation	Addition	nmole 5' GMP formed/min/ mg protein	
		Light	Dark
Bovine retina homogenate	None	34.3	8.7
Bovine retina homogenate	Bleached rhodopsin	33.8	32.6
Bovine retina homogenate	Unbleached rhodopsin	33.9	14.5
Bovine rod outer segments	Unbleached rhodopsin	162	151
Bovine rod outer segments	Bleached rhodopsin	151	148

Further experiments were designed to ascertain that the phosphodiesterase stimulation observed was indeed dependent on rhodopsin bleaching. Suspensions of purified rhodopsin were illuminated till 80 percent bleaching had occurred; rhodopsin not exposed to light served as control. Aliquots (30 μg protein) of bleached or unbleached suspensions were now added to the phosphodiesterase assay mixture. There was no effect on retinal phosphodiesterase activity in the _light_ (Table 2.4). Addition of the bleached preparation, however, increased the _dark_ activity almost up to the activity determined in the _light_. The light stimulation can thus be mimicked by adding bleached rhodopsin preparations free of phosphodiesterase activity. The stimulatory action of these preparations cannot have been due to traces of dodecylsulfate, since low concentrations of the detergent inhibited rather than activated retinal phosphodiesterase activity.

Table 2.5. Light stimulation of retinal cyclic GMP phosphodiesterase at several steps of isolation of the rod outer segments

	nmole 5' GMP/min/mg protein	
Fraction	dark	light
total homogenate	12.9	27.4
2000xg supernatant	19.1	45.1
25,000xg supernatant	5.1	9.5
25,000xg pellet	135	142

Outer segments were purified from dark-adapted calf retina as described by Virmaux et al. (1971). Since the phosphate buffer used routinely has an inhibiting effect on phosphodiesterase activity, it was replaced by 10 mM imidazol buffer (pH 7.0) containing 0.1 M NaCl (Busch et al., 1972). During the initial stages of the purification aliquots were taken and assayed for cyclic GMP phosphodiesterase activity in diffuse room light or complete darkness.

In the experiments described before the high phosphodiesterase activity of isolated rod outer segments did not appear to be light-regulated (Tables 2.3 and 2.4). An endogenous soluble factor which is lost during rod outer segment isolation seems to be required for expression of the light-effect. The magnitude of phosphodiesterase activation in crude homogenates was dependent on protein concentration. Diluting the homogenate gradually decreased the stimulation. When aliquots were taken during several steps of outer segment isolation and assayed for phosphodiesterase activity in dark or light, the light stimulation was lost at a stage where a soluble fraction was separated from the bulk of the photoreceptors. The supernatant containing broken off photoreceptor membranes retained its light-sensitivity (Table 2.5). The soluble factor could be ATP, since Miki et al. (1973) have shown that the cyclic nucleotide hydrolysis in purified frog rods can be stimulated by illumination in the presence of ATP. Using our system of adding bleached rhodopsin suspensions, we obtained essentially the same stimulation of bovine rod phosphodiesterase when we added 1 mM ATP to the incubation mixture (Table 2.6). In this system, cyclic AMP and cyclic GMP hydrolysis were stimulated about equally, indicating that the effect of light on cyclic AMP degradation in whole retina homogenates was masked by the presence of a cyclic AMP phos-

Table 2.6. Activation of rod outer segment cyclic nucleotide phosphodiesterase by rhodopsin preparations in the presence of ATP

Addition	With 1 mM ATP		Without ATP	
	nmole 5' GMP/ min/mg protein	% control	nmole 5' GMP/ min/mg protein	% control
None	91	100	63	100
Dark-kept rhodopsin	128	140	48	76
Bleached rhodopsin	362	400	59	94

Rod outer segments were purified from cattle retinae using the technique of Akhtar et al. (1968) and aliquots of the suspensions (50 μg protein) assayed in the dark with 1 mM cyclic GMP as substrate. Aliquots (20 μg protein) of purified rhodopsin suspensions were added to the assay mixture. The protein contributed by the rhodopsin suspension was not taken into account for calculation of specific activities.

phodiesterase located elsewhere than in the outer segments. The ATP requirement showed a remarkable lack of specificity, since equimolar concentrations of GTP, ITP and CTP, but not ADP, AMP or pyrophosphate, could effectively replace ATP.

Our rhodopsin preparations contain membrane-bound lipids, among them also retinaldehyde. All-trans retinaldehyde released during bleaching is a possible candidate for the transmission of the stimulatory effect. However, when added in a concentration equivalent to that of the rhodopsin preparations, all-trans retinaldehyde was without effect on retinal cyclic GMP phosphodiesterase. Another substance which could be released upon bleaching is membrane-bound calcium. Rod outer segments contain high concentrations of calcium (see Bonting, this book, ch. 3), hence it is not surprising that addition of calcium did not change either the basal or the light-stimulated enzyme activity. Therefore, we investigated whether the calcium chelating agent EGTA would affect the stimulation of retinal phosphodiesterase by bleached rhodopsin. EGTA was devoid of any effect, when added in a final concentration of 0.2 mM. At 2 mM, the control activity was drastically reduced, but the activity measured in the presence of bleached rhodopsin was not changed (Table 2.7). Thus Ca^{2+} ions could be involved in regulating basal

Table 2.7. Effect of retinaldehyde and EGTA on retinal phosphodiesterase activity and its stimulation by bleached rhodopsin

Addition	5' GMP formed nmole/min/mg protein		
	Control	+ Unbleached rhodopsin	+ Bleached rhodopsin
None	8.6	10.6	33.4
All-trans retinaldehyde 4 μM	6.1	8.8	31.1
EGTA 0.2 mM	10.0	11.8	26.8
EGTA 2 mM	0.7	1.2	34.5

Retina homogenates (0.6 - 0.8 mg protein/assay) were assayed for cyclic GMP phosphodiesterase activity (substrate concentration 1 mM) in the dark. EGTA was incubated with the homogenate for 1 hr at 0°C, all-trans retinaldehyde was added directly to the assay mixture. Aliquots (30 μg) of unbleached or 80% bleached rhodopsin suspensions were added to the phosphodiesterase assay.

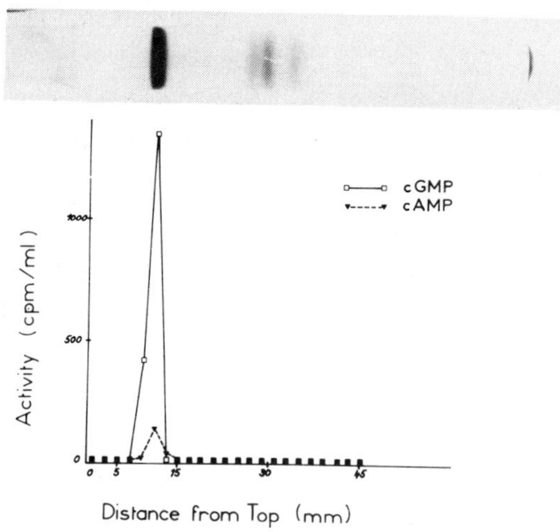

Fig. 2.2. Gel electrophoresis of purified rod outer segment phosphodiesterase. The staining profile (Coomassie brilliant blue) is shown in the upper part; below the activity profile after elution from 2 mm-gel slices is given using 1 μM cyclic nucleotide as substrate.

Table 2.8. Extraction of cyclic GMP phosphodiesterase from bovine rod outer segments

	nmole 5' GMP formed/min/ mg protein	Percent recovered activity
Rod outer segments	42.2	---
1st wash	312.4	73.2
2nd wash	226.6	17.1
Remaining pellet	4.0	9.7

Packed rod outer segments (10 mg of protein) were homogenized in 5 ml of 10 mM Tris-HCl (pH 7.2) and the membranes sedimented (1 h at 10^5 x g). The pellet was washed once with 5 ml of the same buffer. Of the activity originally present 73% was recovered in the 3 fractions. Substrate concentration was 10 μM.

phosphodiesterase activity, but the extent of stimulation by bleached rhodopsin does not seem to be affected.

Most of the phosphodiesterase activity appears in the 10^5 x g supernatant after osmotic shock of the outer segments (Table 2.8). Using this buffer extract as starting material, a highly purified enzyme of high specific activity was obtained. Polyacrylamide gel electrophoresis of the enzyme preparation showed the presence of one major and three minor bands, the enzyme activity being associated with the major band (Fig. 2.2). The enzyme eluted from the gel columns was still able to hydrolyze cyclic GMP and cyclic AMP. At all substrate concentrations tested, cyclic GMP was hydrolyzed at least 20 times faster than cyclic AMP. When the enzyme which had been eluted from polyacrylamide gels was re-electrophoresed in the presence of 0.1 percent sodium dodecylsulfate, a single protein band was obtained.

The enzyme showed anomalous kinetic behaviour: the plot of reaction velocity against substrate concentration was hyperbolic at low (<3 μM) and sigmoidal at higher concentrations (Fig. 2.3). Due to the complex kinetics, no estimation of a K_M-value was possible. Upon storage of the enzyme at $+4^oC$, the kinetic behaviour changed gradually, approaching Michaelis-Menten kinetics. After several days, the intermediary plateau of the saturation plot had

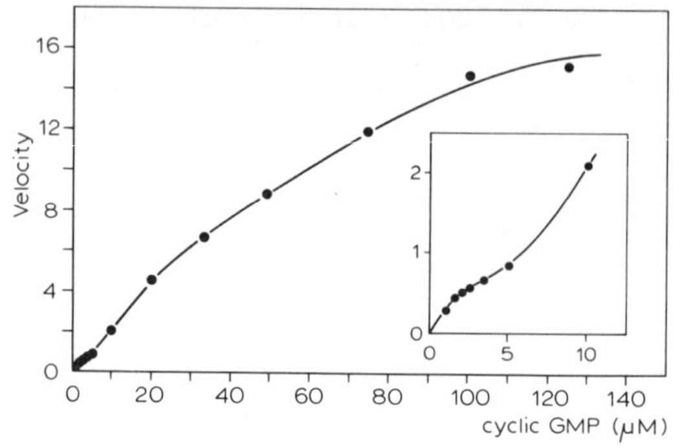

Fig. 2.3. Saturation plot of cyclic GMP hydrolysis by purified rod outer segment phosphodiesterase. The unit of velocity is pmole/min/μl enzyme preparation. The smaller panel shows in expanded scale the velocities for substrate levels up to 10 μM.

disappeared. This shift of the kinetics was accompanied by an increase of enzymatic activity; in the case of the preparation depicted in Fig. 2.3, the specific activity increased from 2.1 to 4.6 μmole GMP formed/min/mg protein (with 10 μM cyclic GMP as substrate) in the course of one week. In spite of the instability of the kinetic characteristics, the deviation from normal kinetics could be reproduced with three different enzyme preparations. With cyclic AMP as substrate, fresh or aged preparations displayed normal kinetic behaviour with an apparent K_M of 0.1 mM. Plots of reaction velocity against substrate concentration such as found for cyclic GMP hydrolysis with freshly purified photoreceptor enzyme resemble the curves analyzed by Teipel and Koshland (1969). Following their interpretation, such curves can be obtained if (1) in a mixture of two proteins one shows classical Michaelis-Menten or negatively cooperative kinetics and the other one positively cooperative kinetics; (2) in the case of a single protein the substrate induces conformational changes which lead to negative cooperativity at low and positive cooperativity at high concentrations. We tend to favour the second possibility since a single peak of enzymatic activity was obtained upon polyacrylamide gel electrophoresis. A phosphodiesterase showing negative cooperativity at low and positive cooperativity at higher concentrations might be physiologically important for the regulation of photoreceptor cyclic GMP levels. At low concentrations (below around 2 μM), the negatively cooperative kinetics will favour an increase in cyclic GMP levels. The sigmoidal shape of the velocity vs. substrate-concentration plot at higher concentrations will prevent a further rise. Clearly, cyclic nucleotide phosphodiesterase from rod outer segments shows the properties of a regulatory enzyme with cyclic GMP but not with cyclic AMP as substrate.

The phosphodiesterase activity in the buffer extracts and the purified enzyme were still stimulated by suspensions of bleached rhodopsin, but the specificity of the effect was lost: now, bleached and dark-kept rhodopsin were equally effective. The same effect was seen with and without addition of ATP. A biphasic effect of ATP on phosphodiesterase activity in intact light-exposed rod outer segments has been reported (Miki et al., 1973; Chader et al., 1974b). No such effect on our purified enzyme preparation could be detected when ATP was added in concentrations from 10^{-10} to 10^{-3}M.

The experimental data point to outer segment phosphodiesterase as the main site for light-regulation of the cyclic GMP levels in photoreceptor cells. Work from several laboratories (Miki et al., 1973; Goridis and Virmaux, 1974; Chader et al., 1974b; Keirns et al., 1975; Goridis et al., 1975) has elucidated some features of the light-activation of this enzyme, but we still do not understand the underlying mechanism in molecular terms. The fact that illumination can be mimicked by adding purified bleached rhodopsin and the availability of a highly purified enzyme will certainly facilitate the search for the effectors involved in the light-stimulation.

The importance of cyclic nucleotide phosphodiesterase for the structural integrity of the photoreceptor cells is underlined by the observation that deficiency of this enzyme precedes rod degeneration in the C3H mouse retina (Schmidt and Lolley, 1973). A concomitant increase of the cyclic GMP levels in the photoreceptor layer has been found (Farber and Lolley, 1974). It was suggested that the presence of high levels of this nucleotide might be responsible for the observed degeneration.

LIGHT-STIMULATED PROTEIN KINASE OF ROD OUTER SEGMENTS: LACK OF EFFECT OF CYCLIC NUCLEOTIDES

It is now well established that many of the diverse actions of cyclic AMP are mediated through regulation of the state of phosphorylation of specific proteins. For cyclic GMP, stimulation of the phosphorylation of endogenous

Table 2.9. The effect of phosphodiesterase inhibitors and cyclic nucleotides on the intrinsic protein kinase activity of rod outer segments

Phosphodiesterase inhibitor	Cyclic nucleotide	Percent control dark	Percent control light
SQ 20 009		95 ± 5	61 ± 2
SQ 20 009	Cyclic AMP 1 mM	91 ± 5	59 ± 4
SQ 20 009	Cyclic GMP 0.1 mM	102	56 ± 4
Theophylline		86 ± 13	62 ± 7
Theophylline	Cyclic AMP 1 mM	99 ± 1	62 ± 6
Theophylline	Cyclic GMP 0.1 mM	n.d.	60, 70
Papaverine		106 ± 5	89 ± 8
Papaverine	Cyclic AMP 1 mM	114 ± 27	79 ± 12
Papaverine	Cyclic GMP 0.1 mM	n.d.	85, 91
Papaverine	Cyclic AMP 1 mM	104 ± 9	95 ± 8
Papaverine	Cyclic GMP 0.1 mM	98 ± 8	93 ± 5
Papaverine	Dibutyryl cyclic AMP 1 mM	99 ± 12	77 ± 12
Papaverine	Dibutyryl cyclic GMP 1 mM	99 ± 16	103 ± 4

Phosphorylation of rod outer segment membrane protein by endogenous protein kinase was measured as described by Weller et al. (1975) in the light or in the dark with the additions indicated. The concentration of SQ 20,009 was 1 mM, of theophylline 10 mM and of papaverine 2 mM. Results are means ± S.D. for 4 - 10 experiments. The activity without addition was set at 100%. (From Weller et al., 1975).

protein has also been described (Casnellie and Greengard, 1974). However, so far it is uncertain whether or not this cyclic nucleotide functions by regulating protein phosphorylation. Rod outer segments have been shown to contain a protein kinase activity which phosphorylates rhodopsin in a light-stimulated reaction (Bownds et al., 1972; Kühn and Dreyer, 1972; Frank et al., 1973; Kühn et al., 1973; Weller et al., 1975; Miller and Paulsen, 1975). Therefore, we have designed experiments to determine whether this kinase activity might be controlled by cyclic nucleotides, in particular by cyclic GMP.

Table 2.10. Inhibition of cyclic nucleotide phosphodiesterase activity from rod outer segments by various inhibitors

Substrate	Phosphodiesterase activity percent control		
	Theophylline 10 mM	SQ 20 009 1 mM	Papaverine 2 mM
Cyclic GMP 10 μM	55	4	5
Cyclic GMP 1 mM	72	12	14
Cyclic AMP 10 μM	58	8	11
Cyclic AMP 1 mM	76	18	21

Suspensions of rod outer segments (50 μg of protein) were pre-incubated with the inhibitors for 10 min at 0°C. The activity of untreated controls was set at 100 percent.

Since rod outer segments contain high phosphodiesterase activity, we have used the phosphodiesterase inhibitors theophylline, SQ 20,009 (which is structurally similar to theophylline) and papaverine. We found that theophylline and SQ 20,009 are both strong inhibitors of outer segment phosphorylation (Table 2.9). This effect was not shared by papaverine, which at the concentrations employed is much more effective as phosphodiesterase inhibitor than theophylline (Table 2.10). Addition of the cyclic nucleotides or their derivatives did not enhance the effect of the phosphodiesterase inhibitors. When added alone, only dibutyryl cyclic AMP slightly reduced the phosphate incorporation (Table 2.9). Since in these experiments whole rod outer segments were used, it may have been difficult for the cyclic nucleotides to reach the kinase inside the rods. To solve this problem, we have used a partially purified system consisting of soluble protein kinase and suspensions of purified rhodopsin. The enzyme responsible for the phosphorylation of rhodopsin can readily be extracted from the outer segments by osmotic shock (Weller et al. 1975) and will phosphorylate purified bleached rhodopsin. The rate of phosphorylation of intact light-exposed outer segments was essentially the same as the rate at which the buffer extract phosphorylated purified bleached rhodopsin, when the two were recombined in the same proportion as in the intact material. Like with intact rod outer segments, theophylline and

Table 2.11. The effect of phosphodiesterase inhibitors and cyclic nucleotides on the protein kinase activity of buffer extracts of rod outer segments

Inhibitor	Cyclic nucleotide (0.1 mM)	Percent of control activity
SQ 20 009 1 mM	---	20 ± 2
SQ 20 009 1 mM	cAMP	18 ± 3.1
SQ 20 009 1 mM	cGMP	17.5 ± 3.2
theophylline 10 mM	-	51.5 ± 6.3
theophylline 10 mM	cAMP	50.7 ± 4.1
theophylline 10 mM	cGMP	50.3 ± 1.9
papaverine 2 mM	-	88.3 ± 6.4
papaverine 2 mM	cAMP	75.5 ± 7.5
papaverine 2 mM	cGMP	82.7 ± 4.7
-	cAMP	101 ± 2.4
-	cGMP	102 ± 3.6
-	Dibut cGMP	100, 97
-	Dibut cAMP	98 ± 2
-	8-Br-cGMP	97 ± 4

Incubations were carried out for 2 min in white light with 200 μg/ml of rhodopsin and 25 - 32 μg/ml of Tris-extracted protein, using 1 mM ATP as phosphate donor in the presence of 5 mM $MgCl_2$. Results are shown as means ± S.D. for 4 - 6 experiments. The activity without additions was set at 100 percent.

SQ 20,009 were strongly inhibitory to the phosphorylation of purified rhodopsin, while cyclic GMP or cyclic AMP alone or in the presence of phosphodiesterase inhibitors had no effect (Table 2.11). Since in this system endogenous cyclic nucleotides are not present, the effect of theophylline or SQ 20,009 must be due to a direct inhibition of protein kinase activity. Essentially the same results are obtained when GTP instead of ATP is used as phosphate donor.

The results are in agreement with those of other workers (Kühn and Dreyer, 1972; Frank et al., 1973), who without giving experimental details reported that the phosphorylation of outer segments is unaffected by cyclic AMP.

Table 2.12. Lack of effect of cyclic nucleotides on rod outer segment phosphatase activity

Papaverine (2 mM)	Cyclic nucleotide (0.1 mM)	Percentage of bound phosphate lost
-	-	14 ± 4
-	cGMP	13 ± 3
-	cAMP	12 ± 5
-	8-bromo-cGMP	10 ± 5
+	-	11 ± 3
+	cAMP	14 ± 4
+	cGMP	12 ± 3

Samples of outer segments were bleached by exposure to white light and then incubated with 1 mM $MgCl_2$, 1 mM [^{32}P]ATP and 50 mM Tris-HCl (pH 7.4) at a protein concentration of 0.4 mg/ml for 30 min at 37°C. The suspension was then centrifuged at 100,000 g for 10 min and washed twice by resuspension and centrifugation from 50 mM sodium phosphate buffer (pH 7.0) to remove noncovalently bound phosphate. The phosphorylated preparation was then incubated in dim red light at 37°C at a concentration of 0.25 mg of protein/ml with 50 mM Tris HCl (pH 7.4), 2 mM $MgCl_2$ and the stated concentration of cyclic nucleotide or phosphodiesterase inhibitor. Samples were taken at zero time or after 20 min and the amount of bound radioactive phosphate determined.
Results are shown as means ± S.D. for 4 experiments.

Pannbacker and Schoch (1973) and Pannbacker (1974), however, have reported that rod outer segments contain a soluble protein kinase activity which phosphorylates histones in a cyclic AMP stimulated reaction. The kinase activity containing extracts in our experiments showed slight if any activity towards histones, which was unaffected by cyclic AMP (Weller et al., 1975). As pointed out above, recombination experiments give no indication that intact rods contain a protein kinase activity other than that found in the buffer-extracts.

In toad bladder, cyclic AMP controls the state of protein phosphorylation by regulating not protein kinase but protein phosphatase activity (De Lorenzo et al., 1973). Rod outer segments contain an enzyme which cleaves the phosphate from the rhodopsin molecule (Frank et al, 1973; Kühn et al., 1973; Weller et

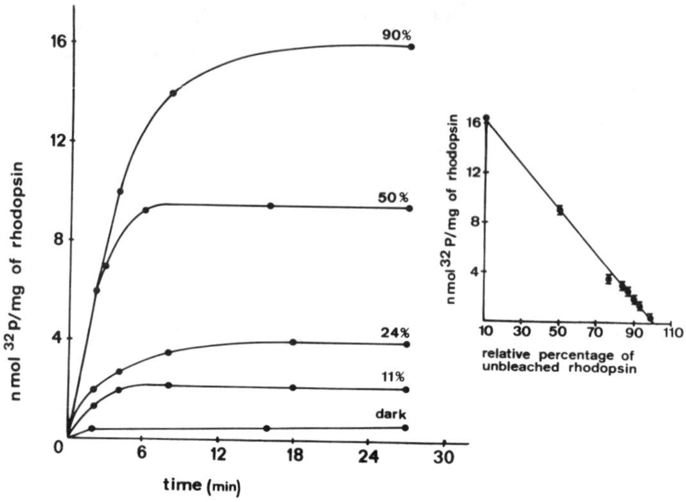

Fig. 2.4. The effect of bleaching on the phosphorylation of rhodopsin. Samples of purified rhodopsin were bleached to various extents by exposure to white light and the extent of bleaching estimated by measuring the decrease in absorbance at 500 nm. The time-course of phosphorylation was determined in dim red light. In the smaller panel, the maximal phosphate incorporation in partially bleached rhodopsin is plotted against the percentage of bleaching. (From Weller et al., 1975).

al., 1975). However, this activity is not influenced by cyclic nucleotides (Table 2.12).

If the phosphorylation of rod outer segments is not controlled by cyclic nucleotides, how can light stimulate phosphate incorporation? We again took advantage of the partially purified system using a buffer-extract as enzyme source and purified rhodopsin as substrate. The Tris-extract catalyzes the phosphorylation of purified photobleached rhodopsin, but not of unbleached rhodopsin (Fig. 2.4). Exposure of the buffer-extract to light did not cause it to phosphorylate unbleached rhodopsin, neither did it affect the rate at which it catalyzed the phosphorylation of bleached rhodopsin. The Tris-extract thus contains a protein kinase which is not affected by light but which catalyzes the phosphorylation of bleached rhodopsin. If purified rhodopsin is bleached to different degrees, the more highly bleached preparations can be more readily phosphorylated (in dim red light) with opsin kinase. Both the initial rate of phosphorylation and the total amount of phosphate which can be incorporated are increased (Fig. 2.4). When the amount of phosphate, which can be maximally incorporated into the rhodopsin in the sample, is plotted against the percentage of unbleached rhodopsin, a completely linear relationship is found (Fig. 2.4). Apparently, the amount of phosphate which can be incorporated into a sample of rhodopsin is directly proportional to the number of molecules of bleached rhodopsin. Light thus stimulates the phosphorylation of rhodopsin in intact outer segments by increasing the amount of substrate (bleached rhodopsin) available to the kinase. Since the illuminated rhodopsin suspensions can be stored at $4^{o}C$ for any period of time without losing the property of being phosphorylated, it is highly unlikely that a photoproduct of rhodopsin other than opsin is preferentially phosphorylated.

LIGHT-INDUCED CHANGES OF THE ENDOGENOUS CYCLIC GMP CONTENT OF INTACT RETINA

If cyclic GMP were to play a role in visual excitation, light should exert a rapid and drastic effect on its concentration in the photoreceptor cells. The outer segments depend on the inner segments for the supply of nucleotide triphosphates (Cohen, 1963) and the endogenous nucleotide metabolism cannot be studied in the isolated organelles. Only enzymatic activities can be measured in purified rods. By contrast, an active nucleotide metabolism has been shown to persist in isolated retinae for several hours (Urban, 1972) and retinae, incubated in a physiological medium, are capable of synthetizing [^{3}H]cyclic GMP from tritiated hypoxanthine (Goridis and Virmaux, 1974). High cyclic GMP concentrations were found in intact bovine retinae incubated in a physiological medium (64 pmole/mg protein, S.E. 3 for N = 11). During illumination there was a pronounced and rapid drop of retinal cyclic GMP levels. When diffuse, dim room light (200 lux at the level of the incubation vessels) was present for only 15 sec before stopping the final incubation, cyclic GMP concentrations decreased by 70 percent. Even light exposure for only 5 sec caused a 30 percent drop of the cyclic GMP content (Fig. 2.5).

In vivo rods are functional only at light intensities which bleach a small percentage of their rhodopsin content and physiological significance can only be attributed to those reactions which are influenced by light intensities within the normal working range of the rod cell. Moreover, since maximum physiological responses are obtained when bleaching of rhodopsin is

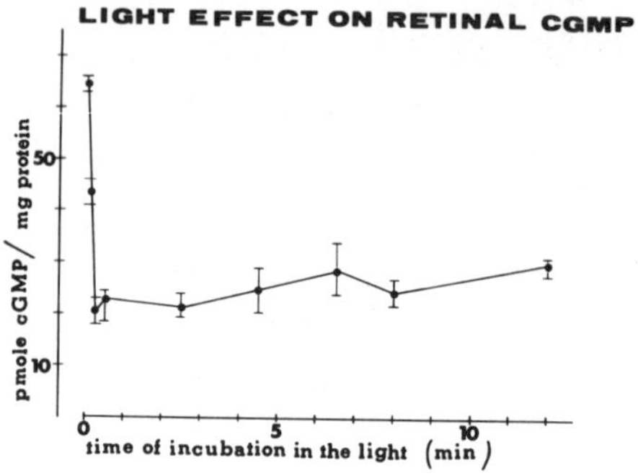

Fig. 2.5. The effect of light exposure on cyclic GMP concentrations in intact calf retina. Diffuse fluorescent room light was present during incubation. Cyclic GMP concentrations are given as the mean ± the range for 2 - 3 experiments. The first point represents the non-illuminated controls, given as mean ± S.E. for 11 experiments. (From Goridis et al., 1974).

negligible, these low levels of illumination should give a maximal effect on chemical events involved in this response. In bovine retinae, obtained from animals which had not been dark-adapted before slaughter, some of the rhodopsin is already in the bleached state. Therefore, we used retinae of fully dark-adapted frogs which were mounted in a small superfusion chamber and were then illuminated by a flashlight. Here again light provoked a drastic drop of

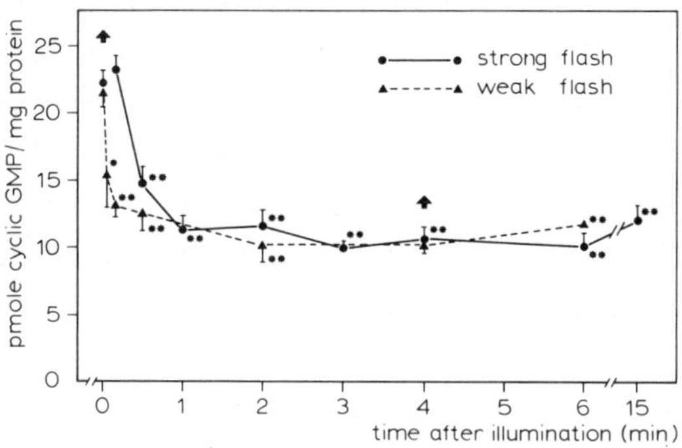

Fig. 2.6. The effect of flash-illumination on cyclic GMP concentrations in intact frog retinae. Δ designates experiments where 10 mM sodium aspartate was added to the superfusion medium; the weak flash was used. The mean ±S.E. is given for 4 to 12 experiments, except where only two experiments had been performed and the average value is given. An asterisk designates values significantly different from dark-levels (* $p< 0.05$, ** $p< 0.005$).

retinal cyclic GMP concentrations (Fig. 2.6). The same maximal response was elicited by a bright and by a weak flash-light, the decrease of the cyclic GMP concentrations being 55 and 53 percent,respectively. By comparison with a fully dark-adapted control, the amount of rhodopsin bleached by the weaker flash was below the limit of the sensitivity of our recordings, that is less than 5 percent of the rhodopsin was in the bleached state. Apparently, endogenous cyclic GMP levels are maximally influenced by low light intensities which are within or near the physiological working range of the rod cells. In agreement with these results, Keirns et al. (1975) reported that cyclic nucleotide phosphodiesterase in isolated outer segments was activated in the presence of very low concentrations of bleached rhodopsin. The drop of cyclic GMP levels was slower after the bright than after the weak stimulus: no significant response was observed 10 sec after a strong flash, minimal values being attained after 1 min, whereas the weaker stimulus provoked a significant fall of cyclic GMP levels in only 3 sec and a nearly maximal response was observed after 30 sec. At present, we cannot explain this difference in the kinetics of the response. Certainly, the bleaching produced by the strong flash is unphysiological for rod photoreceptor cells.

Since whole retinae have been used in these experiments we could not tell whether the observed changes were occurring in the rod cells or elsewhere in the retina. Several lines of evidence, however, indicate that this change is in fact occurring in the photoreceptor cells. As pointed out above, about 90 percent of retinal guanylate cyclase activity is associated with the outer segments and highly purified outer segments contain a phosphodiesterase activity stimulated by light or bleached rhodopsin (Miki et al., 1973; Keirns et al., 1975; Goridis et al., 1975). Moreover, also in intact retinae evidence supporting a photoreceptor localisation of the effect was obtained. Such rapid effects as the drop of cyclic GMP content can be assumed to be transmitted to other retinal structures via nerve impulses. Sodium aspartate has been shown to uncouple the electrical activity of the photoreceptor cells from the inner retinal layers (Penn and Hagins, 1969; Sillman et al., 1969a). An essentially unchanged response to a weak flash was obtained when 10 mM aspartate was included in the superfusion fluid (Fig. 2.6, Δ).

In some cases, cyclic AMP has been determined along with cyclic GMP on the same samples. Considerably lower cyclic AMP concentrations were found in frog

Table 2.13. Effect of flash-illumination on retinal cyclic nucleotide levels

Time after illumination	Cyclic AMP	Cyclic GMP
	pmole/mg protein	
0 (control)	5.06 ± 0.11	25.0 ± 0.4
10 sec	4.81 ± 0.21^x	12.2 ± 0.6 *
60 sec	4.83 ± 0.16^x	14.4 ± 0.7 *

The mean ± S.E. is shown for 3 experiments
$^x p > 0.2$ $\quad$ $*p < 0.01$

retinae, and these were not influenced by light (Table 2.13). Retinal adenylate cyclase appears to be enriched in inner retinal structures as compared with rod outer segments (Hendriks et al., 1973; Manthorpe and McConnell, 1974). By microdissection of the retina considerably lower cyclic AMP concentrations are found in a photoreceptor-enriched layer than in whole retina (Lolley et al., 1974). Therefore, our results do not exclude the possibility that moderate changes of cyclic AMP concentrations occurring in the rod cells were masked by the higher cyclic AMP content of the rest of the retina. In any case, cyclic GMP appears to be the cyclic nucleotide specifically involved in photoreceptor function.

CONCLUSIONS

Considerable evidence has accumulated recently which points to cyclic GMP as an important intermediate in visual excitation although its precise function is unclear at present. The two most likely functions of cyclic GMP are:
(1) cyclic GMP serves as the "internal transmitter" linking photon capture by the rhodopsin molecule to plasma membrane conductivity changes; (2) cyclic GMP assumes a function in the modulation of photoreceptor excitability, i.e. in light- or dark-adaptation. Severe time constraints have to be met, if the drop of cyclic GMP should actually serve as the signal linking rhodopsin bleaching to changes of the sodium influx into the outer segment since the membrane conductivity changes are known to occur in the millisecond-range after illumination. In two systems investigated (dim, constant room light and incubated

cattle retinae, weak flash illumination of superfused frog retinae) significant changes of the cyclic GMP content were seen at the earliest time points, at 5 and 3 sec, respectively. More sophisticated techniques are needed to render measurements in the sub-second range feasible. Clearly, maximum responses are not yet attained after the shortest time intervals. For that reason, and in analogy to the rather slow effect of cyclic nucleotides on the excitability of post-ganglionic sympathetic neurons (Greengard et al., 1972), cerebellar Purkinje cells (Hoffer et al., 1972) and cortical neurons (Stone et al., 1975), we tend to favour the second possibility namely that cyclic GMP acts as regulator of photoreceptor sensitivity.

Definite proof or disproof of a specific function of cyclic GMP can only be obtained by studying the physiological responses of the retinal rod to the addition of exogenous cyclic GMP, its analogues or of phosphodiesterase inhibitors. Effects of cyclic AMP or its dibutyryl derivative on the *Limulus* eye receptor potential have been reported (Miller et al., 1971; Wulff, 1971), but AMP can produce similar effects (Wulff, 1973). Other studies have been hampered by the fact that the phosphodiesterase inhibitors used are rather ineffective against outer segment phosphodiesterase (see Table 2.10) or are also inhibitory to rhodopsin phosphorylation (see Table 2.11). Ebrey and Hood (1973), however, used the more potent phosphodiesterase inhibitor papaverine, which does not affect rhodopsin phosphorylation, in addition to theophylline, SQ 20,006 and caffeine. The only effect common to all phosphodiesterase inhibitors, and the only one seen with papaverine, was a decrease of the amplitude of the receptor potential when the retina was dark-adapted. The authors conclude that cyclic AMP can cause the rods to be filled with sodium ions in the dark, possibly by increasing the dark-permeability of the membrane envelope. Hood and Ebrey (1974) linked their results to changes of cyclic *AMP* levels brought about by phosphodiesterase inhibition. It follows from our results that cyclic *GMP* should be examined.

Our results clearly demonstrate that the phosphorylation and dephosphorylation of rhodopsin are not regulated by cyclic GMP. In agreement with other authors (Kühn and Dreyer, 1972; Frank et al., 1973) we do not detect phosphorylation of any outer segment protein other than rhodopsin. Yet we cannot exclude that a minor protein constituent, e.g. of the outer membrane envelope, might be phosphorylated in a cyclic GMP dependent reaction. Also the remote

Table 2.14. Occurrence of cyclic GMP in the bathing medium of incubated frog retina

	pmole cyclic GMP	
	Medium	Tissue
Light	3.4 ± 0.42	18 ± 1.4
Dark	0.97± 0.11	34 ± 2.9

Retinae of dark-adapted Ranae esculentae were used. After 30 min pre-incubation in modified frog Ringer (see Fig. 2.6), the retinae were transferred into fresh medium (2 retinae in 1 ml) and incubated at room temperature for 10 min in diffuse room light or dim red light. At the end of the incubation period, the retinae were removed with a forceps and dropped into 1 M $HClO_4$. The medium was rapidly filtered through Millipore (0.45 μ) filters into 0.1 ml 7 M $HClO_4$ and the cyclic GMP content determined after neutralisation. The results are expressed as pmole cyclic GMP/2 retinae or 1 ml medium; the mean ± S.E. is shown for three experiments.

possibility should be considered that cyclic GMP is extruded from the outer segments and acts elsewhere than in the rods, e.g. in the pigment epithelium, which shows light-dependent migration of pigment granules (Ali, 1971). We found low but measurable levels of cyclic GMP in the medium of incubated frog retinae which were higher in the light than in the dark (Table 2.14); but the cyclic GMP secreted over a 10 min period represented only 2.8 percent of the amount recovered within the tissue in darkness and 19 percent in light.

The function of sensory receptors bears important similarities to synaptic transmission; in both events, conformational changes of membrane-bound macromolecules have to be translated into a signal, which can be transported and processed by nerve cells, that is into membrane conductivity changes. In the function of sensory receptors as in synaptic transmission, the rapid generation of a nervous impulse and slower changes of the excitability can be differentiated. Elucidation of the precise function of cyclic GMP in the rod cells will therefore contribute to our understanding of the role of this cyclic nucleotide in synaptic transmission.

REFERENCES

Akhtar M., Blosse P.T. and Dewhurst P.B. (1968) The nature of the retinal-opsin linkage. Biochem. J. 110, 693-698

Ali M.A. (1971) Les réponses rétinomotrices: Caractères et mécanismes. Vision Res. 11, 1225-1288

Bensinger R.E., Fletcher R.T. and Chader G.J. (1974) Guanylate cyclase: inhibition by light in retinal photoreceptors. Science 183, 86-87

Bitensky M.W., Gorman R.E. and Miller W.H. (1971) Adenyl cyclase as a link between photon capture and changes in membrane permeability of frog photoreceptors. Proc. Acad. Sci. USA 68, 561-562

Bownds D., Dawes J., Miller J. and Stahlman M. (1972) Phosphorylation of frog photoreceptor membranes induced by light. Nature new biology 237, 125-127

Bownds D., Brodic A., Robinson W.E., Palmer D., Miller J. and Shedlovsky A. (1974) Physiology and enzymology of frog photoreceptor membranes. Exp. Eye Res. 18, 253-269

Busch G.E., Appleburg M.L., Lamola P.M. and Rentzepis P.M. (1972) Formation and decay of pre-lumirhodopsin at room temperature. Proc. Nat. Acad. Sci. USA 69, 2802-2806

Cailla H.L., Racine-Weisbuch M.S. and Delaage M.A. (1973) Cyclic AMP assay at 10^{-15}mole level. Analyt. Biochem. 56, 394-407

Cailla H.L., Vannier C.J. and Delaage M.A. (1975) Guanosine 3'5' cyclic monophosphate assay at 10^{-15}mole level. Analyt. Biochem. (in press)

Casnellie J.E. and Greengard P. (1974) Cyclic GMP-dependent phosphorylation of endogenous substrate proteins in membranes of mammalian smooth muscle. Proc. Nat. Acad. Sci. USA 71, 1891-1895

Chader G.J., Johnson M., Fletcher R.T. and Bensinger R.E. (1974a) Cyclic nucleotide phosphodiesterase of the bovine retina: Activity, subcellular distribution and kinetic parameters. J. Neurochem. 22, 93-99

Chader G.J., Fletcher R., Johnson M. and Bensinger R. (1974b) Rod outer segment phosphodiesterase: factors affecting the hydrolysis of cyclic AMP and cyclic GMP. Exp. Eye Res. 18, 509-515

Cohen A.J. (1963) Vertebrate retinal cells and their organisation. Biological Reviews 38, 427-459

Cohen A.J. (1970) Further studies on the question of the patency of saccules in outer segments of vertebrate photoreceptors. Vision Res. 10, 445-453

Cone R.A. and Pak W.L. (1971) The early receptor potential. In: Handbook of Sensory Physiology, Vol. 1 (Loewenstein W.R. ed.) pp. 345-365, Springer Berlin

Coquil J.F., Virmaux N., Mandel P. and Goridis C. (1975) Cyclic nucleotide phosphodiesterase of retinal photoreceptors. Partial purification and some properties of the enzyme. Biochim. Biophys. Acta 403, 425-437

De Lorenzo R.J., Walton K.G., Curran P.F. and Greengard P. (1973) Regulation of phosphorylation of a specific protein in toad bladder by ADH and cyclic AMP and its possible relationship to membrane permeability changes. Proc. Nat. Acad. Sci. USA 70, 880-884

Ebrey T.G. and Hood D.C. (1973) The effects of cyclic nucleotide phosphodiesterase inhibitors on the frog rod receptor potential. In: Biochemistry and Physiology of Visual Pigments (Langer H. ed.) pp. 341-348, Springer Berlin

Farber D.B. and Lolley, R.W. (1974) Cyclic guanosine monophosphate: elevation in degenerating photoreceptor cells of the C3H mouse retina. Science 186, 449-451

Frank R.W., Cavannagh H.D. and Kenyon K.R. (1973) Light-stimulated phosphorylation of bovine visual pigments by ATP. J. Biol. Chem. 248, 596-608

Goridis C. and Morgan I.G. (1973) Guanyl cyclase in rat brain subcellular fractions. Febs Letters 34, 71-73

Goridis C., Virmaux N., Urban P.F. and Mandel P. (1973) Guanyl cyclase in a mammalian photoreceptor. Febs Letters 30, 163-166

Goridis C. and Virmaux N. (1974) Light regulated guanosine 3'5' monophosphate phosphodiesterase of bovine retina. Nature 248, 57-58

Goridis C., Virmaux N., Cailla H.L. and Delaage M.A. (1974) Rapid light-induced changes of retinal cyclic GMP levels. Febs Letters 49, 167-169

Goridis C. and Reutter W. (1975) Plasma membrane-associated increase of guanylate cyclase activity in regenerating rat liver. Nature 257, 698-700

Goridis C., Virmaux N. Weller M., Coquil J.F. and Mandel P. (1975) Guanylate cyclase and cyclic GMP phosphodiesterase in vertebrate photoreceptor organelles. In: Proceedings of the IXth Congress of the Collegium Internationale Neuropsychopharmacologicum, Paris, 1974 (Boissier J.R., Hippius H. and Pichot P., eds). Excerpta Medica Amsterdam (in press)

Greengard P., McAfee D.A. and Kebabian J.V. (1972) On the mechanism of action of cyclic AMP and its role in synaptic transmission. In: Advances in Cyclic Nucleotide Research, Vol. 1 (Greengard P., Paoletti R. and Robison G.A., eds) pp. 337-355, Raven Press, New-York

Hagins W.A. (1972) The visual process: excitatory mechanisms in the primary receptor cells. Ann. Rev. Biophys. Bioeng. 1, 131-158

Hardman J.G. and Sutherland E.W. (1969) Guanyl cyclase, an enzyme catalyzing the formation of guanosine 3'5'-monophosphate from guanosine triphosphate. J. Biol. Chem. 244, 6363-6370

Helwig J.J., Bollack C., Mandel P. and Goridis C. (1975) Renal cortex guanylate cyclase. Preferential enrichment in glomerular membranes. Biochim. Biophys. Acta 377, 463-471

Hemminki K. (1974) Properties of highly purified retinal outer segments. Vision Res. 14, 551-554

Hendriks T., De Pont J.J.H.H.M., Daemen F.J.M. and Bonting S.L. (1973) Adenylate cyclase and rod photoreceptor membranes: a critical appraisal. Biochim. Biophys. Acta 347, 491-493

Hoffer B.J., Siggins G.R., Oliver A.P. and Bloom F.E. (1972) Cyclic AMP-mediated adrenergic synapses to cerebellar Purkinje cells. In: Advances in Cyclic Nucleotide Research, Vol. 1 (Greengard P., Paoletti R. and Robison G.A., eds) pp. 411-423, Raven Press, New-York

Hood D.C. and Ebrey T.G. (1974) On the possible role of cyclic AMP in dark adaptation. Vision Res. 14, 437-440

Keirns J.J., Miki N., Bitensky M.W. and Keirns M. (1975) A link between rhodopsin and disc membrane cyclic nucleotide phosphodiesterase. Action spectrum and sensitivity to illumination. Biochemistry 14, 2760-2766

Kimura H. and Murad F. (1975) Two forms of guanylate cyclase in mammalian tissues and possible mechanisms for their regulation. Metabolism 24, 439-458

Kühn H. and Dreyer W.J. (1972) Light-dependent phosphorylation of rhodopsin by ATP. Febs Letters 20, 1-6

Kühn H., Cook J.H. and Dreyer W.J. (1973) Phosphorylation of rhodopsin in bovine photoreceptor membranes. A dark reaction after illumination. Biochemistry 12, 2495-2502

Lolley R.N., Schmidt S.Y. and Farber D.B. (1974) Alterations in cyclic AMP metabolism associated with photoreceptor cell degeneration in the C3H mouse. J. Neurochem. 22, 701-707

Manthorpe M. and McConnell D.G. (1974) Adenylate cyclase in vertebrate retina. J. Biol. Chem. 49, 4608-4613

Miki N., Keirns J.J., Marcus F.R., Freeman J. and Bitensky M.W. (1973) Regulation of cyclic nucleotide concentration in photoreceptors: an ATP-dependent stimulation of cyclic nucleotide phosphodiesterase by light. Proc. Nat. Acad. Sci. USA 70, 3820-3824

Miki N., Keirns J.J., Marcus F.R. and Bitensky M.W. (1974) Light-regulation of adenosine 3'5' cyclic monophosphate levels in vertebrate photoreceptors. Exp. Eye Res. 18, 281-297

Miller J.A. and Paulsen R. (1975) Phosphorylation and dephosphorylation of frog rod outer segment membranes as part of the visual process. J. Biol. Chem. 250, 4427-4432

Miller W.H., Gorman R.E. and Bitensky M.W. (1971) Cyclic adenosine monophosphate: function in photoreceptors. Science 174, 295-297

Pannbacker R.G., Fleischman D.E. and Reed D.W. (1972) Cyclic nucleotide phosphodiesterase. High activity in a mammalian photoreceptor. Science 175, 757-758

Pannbacker R.G. (1973) Control of guanylate cyclase activity in the rod outer segment. Science 182, 1138-1140

Pannbacker R.G. and Schoch D.R. (1973) Protein kinases of the rod outer segment. J. Gen. Physiol. 61, 257-258

Pannbacker R.G. (1974) Cyclic nucleotide metabolism in human photoreceptors. Invest. Ophthalmol. 13, 535-538

Penn R.D. and Hagins W.A. (1969) Signal transmission along retinal rods and the origin of the a-wave. Nature 223, 201-208

Schmidt S.Y. and Lolley R.N. (1973) Cyclic nucleotide phosphodiesterase: an early defect in inherited retinal degeneration of C3H mice. J. Cell Biol. 57, 117-123

Schultz G., Böhme E. and Hardman J.G. (1974) Separation and purification of cyclic nucleotides by ion-exchange resin column chromatography. In: Methods in Enzymology, Vol. 38 (Hardman J.G. and O'Malley B., eds). pp. 9-24, Academic Press, New-York

Sillman A.J., Ito H. and Tomita T. (1969a) Studies on the mass receptor potential. I - General Properties. Vision Res. 9, 1435-1442

Sillman A.J., Ito H. and Tomita T. (1969b) Studies on the mass receptor potential of isolated frog retina. II - On the basis of the ionic mechanisms. Vision Res. 9, 1443-1451

Stone T.W., Taylor D.A. and Bloom F.E. (1975) Cyclic AMP and cyclic GMP may mediate opposite neuronal responses in the rat cerebral cortex. Science 187, 845-847

Teipel J. and Koshland D.E. (1969) The significance of intermediary plateau regions. Biochemistry 8, 4656-4663

Thompson W.J. and Appleman M.M. (1971) Multiple cyclic nucleotide phosphodiesterase activities from rat brain. Biochemistry 10, 311-316

Urban P.F. (1972) Contribution à l'étude des mécanismes intervenant au cours de l'excitation visuelle au niveau de la rétine. Thèse de Doctorat ès-Sciences, Université de Strasbourg

Virmaux N., Urban P.F. and Waehnheldt T.V. (1971) Proteins of bovine retinal outer segments: electrophoresis on polyacrylamide gels in the presence of sodium dodecyl sulphate. Febs Letters 12, 325-328

Virmaux N., Waehnheldt T.V. and Urban P.F. (1972) Mise en évidence du changement de conformation de l'opsine, au cours du blanchiment photonique par des études de solubilité dans divers détergents. C.R. Acad. Sci. Paris, D 275, 2041-2044

Virmaux N., Nullans G. and Goridis C. (1975) Guanylate cyclase in vertebrate retina: evidence for specific association with rod outer segments. J. Neurochem. (in press).

Weller M., Virmaux N. and Mandel P. (1975) Light stimulates phosphorylation of rhodopsin in the retina: the presence of a protein kinase that is specific for photobleached rhodopsin. Proc. Nat. Acad. Sci. USA 72, 381-385

White A.A. and Aurbach G.D. (1969) Detection of guanyl cyclase in mammalian tissues. Biochim. Biophys. Acta 191, 686-704

Wulff V.J. (1971) The effect of cyclic AMP on *Limulus* lateral eye retinular cells. Vision Res. 11, 1493-1495

Wulff V.J. (1973) The effect of cyclic AMP and aminophylline on *Limulus* lateral eye retinular cells. Vision Res. 13, 2335-2344

Yoshikami S. and Hagins W.A. (1973) Control of the dark current in vertebrate rods and cones. In: Biochemistry and Physiology of Visual Pigments (Langer H., ed.) pp. 245-255. Springer, New-York

CHAPTER 3

CALCIUM AS A TRANSMITTER IN PHOTORECEPTOR CELLS

S.L. Bonting and F.J.M. Daemen

Dept. of Biochemistry
University of Nijmegen
Nijmegen, The Netherlands

ROD PHOTORECEPTOR EXCITATION

The structure of the rod photoreceptor cell has already been described in Chapter 1 and is shown schematically in Fig. 1.5. The crucial point is that the rod sac membrane, which contains the visual pigment rhodopsin, is separated by a gap of at least 70 Å from the outer membrane of the outer segment. In darkness the latter membrane is highly permeable for sodium ions. This permits a dark current of sodium ions to run along the rod axis from the inner segment to the outer segment, where the sodium ions enter passively. A strong, ouabain-sensitive sodium pump activity in the outer membrane of the inner segment generates this dark current (Hagins, 1972; Tomita, 1972).

Upon illumination a sudden and drastic decrease in the sodium permeability occurs, which leads to hyperpolarization of the outer membrane and a decrease in the dark current. The spreading of the hyperpolarization along the membrane stimulates the rod spherule synapse. Hagins et al (1970) have calculated that the effect is, even at minimal stimulating light intensity, large enough to be noticed over the "dark noise" in the membrane potential.

The electrophysiological evidence for a light-induced decrease in sodium conductance of the outer membrane obtained by Tomita and Hagins and their coworkers has been confirmed by means of rapid osmotic shrinkage measurements on freshly isolated frog outer segments in hypertonic solution (Korenbrot and Cone, 1972). These experiments clearly show that dark-adapted outer segments are permeable for sodium and impermeable for potassium, whereas illumination produces a specific decrease in sodium permeability. Absorption of a single photon per rod is estimated to lower sodium influx by 3%, which would be equivalent to 10^7 sodium ions prevented from entering the outer segment. This means that the actual energy needed for rod excitation is provided by the ATP-driven sodium-pump of the inner segment, whereas the very much smaller energy of a photon is sufficient to trigger the process.

The process is schematically represented in Fig. 3.1: in the dark adapted situation (left) the sodium channels in the outer membrane of the outer segment are open, and the sodium pump in the inner segment generates a large dark current of sodium ions. After illumination (right) a number of sodium

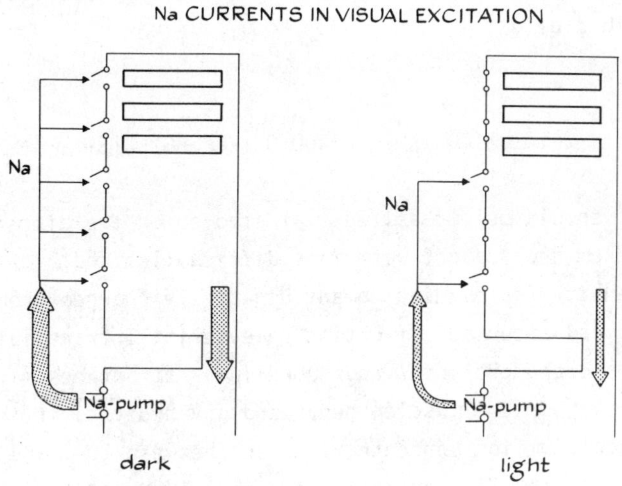

Fig. 3.1. Schematic presentation of the sodium current in the vertebrate rod. In darkness all sodium channels are open, and the current is large. Upon illumination sodium channels close and the current is reduced.

channels have been closed down, leading to a decrease in the dark current.

The crucial question is: how does the change, induced in the rod sac membrane by absorption of a photon, effect the closing of sodium channels in the outer membrane? Further application of his electrophysiological technique has allowed Hagins and his co-workers to establish that increasing the extracellular calcium concentration from 1.4 mM to 20 mM mimics the effect of light on the dark current (Yoshikami and Hagins, 1973). Lowering the extracellular calcium concentration to less than 10^{-7}M severely decreases the light sensitivity of the dark current after 1-2 min. The effects are reversible upon restoring the original calcium level. Application of the ionophore X537A (10^{-5}M) to the external medium decreases the dark current markedly, presumably through increasing the permeability of the outer membrane to calcium (Hagins and Yoshikami, 1974). Their tentative conclusion is that in rods the rod sacs are a store of calcium, which is released in part upon illumination. The released calcium ions would diffuse through the extrasaccular space to the outer membrane, where they would be bound to sodium channels thereby closing them. During dark-adaptation these calcium ions would be reaccumulated by the rod sacs. Experiments aimed at verifying this attractive explanation for the signal transmission from rod sac to outer membrane are described below.

CALCIUM CONTENT OF ROD OUTER SEGMENTS

At the outset it should be emphasized that studies on the distribution and movement of calcium are fraught with many difficulties and pitfalls, mostly due to its propensity for binding to any negatively charged groups. Glassware may bind calcium and after acidification release it! Intracellular compounds (e.g. proteins) and phospholipids and subcellular structures may do so likewise. From previous work on muscle, nerve and erythrocytes it is clear that the cytoplasmic calcium ion concentrations are between 10^{-7} and 10^{-6}M, while the extracellular calcium concentration is about 1 mM and that in sarcoplasmic reticulum and mitochondria may be of the order of 10 mM (Baker, 1972). Maintenance of these gradients requires active calcium pumps. This means that any treatment impairing pump activity, such as cell fractionation procedures, may easily cause large shifts in the intracellular calcium distribution. Hence, extreme caution is needed both in the execution and in the interpretation of experiments.

In order to obtain a supply of fresh outer segments frog retina was used in the earlier experiments (Hendriks et al., 1974). Rana esculenta was found the most suitable species. Outer segments are obtained from the excised retinas of dark adapted animals by gentle shaking for 30 sec in a modified Ringer solution, containing 112 mM NaCl, 3 mM KCl, 3 mM $MgCl_2$, 3 mM ATP, 10 mM glucose, 10 mM Tris-HCl (pH 7.4). The entire procedure, incl. filtration over 60-mesh stainless steel wire screen and centrifugation (2 x 10 min, 1200 x g), takes less than 60 min from the time of death. This method reproducibly yields a suspension containing mainly intact rod outer segments with only minor contamination by mitochondria (myoid body attached to some outer segments) and a few melanin granules (from the pigment epithelium). The yield is highest when ATP is present in the Ringer solution and amounts to nearly half the outer segments present in the retinas, as established by determining rhodopsin according to Hendriks et al. (1973).

Determination by atomic absorption spectroscopy shows the presence of an appreciable amount of calcium, which after two centrifugations is fairly stable upon further washing and centrifugation or upon addition of 10 mM EDTA. Hence, we assume that all calcium present in the sediment after the second centrifugation is located inside the outer segments.

The average calcium content of the outer segment preparations is then 12.4 (S.E.: 0.8, n=38) moles calcium per mol rhodopsin. When ATP is omitted from the Ringer medium during isolation, the calcium content is significantly lower (Table 3.1). Addition of 10 mM EDTA has no effect, indicating that all calcium is sequestered. Sampling of the suspension by means of a constriction micropipette produces a significant loss of calcium, presumably through damaging of outer segments. Therefore, we have always determined calcium in both sediment and supernatant after centrifugation, and have expressed the results as the percentage of calcium which remains in the sediment for each aliquot.

Table 3.1. Calcium content of frog rod outer segments isolated in various ways

Medium	without sampling	with sampling
	moles calcium per mol rhodopsin	
Ringer, 3 mM ATP	12.4 ± 0.8 (38)	8.7 ± 1.5 (13)
Ringer, 3 mM ATP, 10 mM EDTA	12.8 ± 1.6 (4)	8.4 ± 1.6 (3)
Ringer, no ATP, no EDTA	8.0 ± 0.6 (11)	4.6 ± 0.8 (9)

The isolation procedure is described in the text.
Calcium is determined in the sediment after the final centrifugation, and is expressed as moles calcium per mol rhodopsin with the standard error and in parentheses the number of experiments (each in triplicate).
Statistical analysis by means of the Wilcoxon test gives the following P-values:

all values without vs. all values with sampling, $P < 0.001$

all values without vs. all values with EDTA, $P = 0.38$

all values with ATP vs. all values without ATP, $P < 0.001$

Magnesium is also present in rather high concentration in rod outer segments: 1.4 moles magnesium per mol calcium for frog. These concentrations are remarkably high. Assuming a rhodopsin concentration of 2.5 mM in the frog outer segment (Liebman, 1962), the frog would have a calcium concentration of 31 mM over the total outer segment volume. This calcium level is even higher than that in squid axon mitochondria (Baker, 1972), and it should still be higher inside the rod sacs, if nearly all calcium is accumulated there. In a preliminary note Liebman (1974) reports values up to 2 mol calcium per mol rhodopsin in frog rod outer segment preparations; these low values may be due to the way the outer segments have been treated during isolation.

Cattle rod outer segments have also been studied. Since these cannot be isolated by shaking of the retina, the density gradient centrifugation method (De Grip et al, 1972) has been used for their isolation. This is a much more extensive procedure (4 - 6 hrs from time of death). The final suspension in isotonic Tris-HCl buffer contains 2.5 (S.E.: 0.4, n=11) moles calcium per mol rhodopsin (Hendriks, 1975). The much lower calcium level in cattle rod outer segments suggests that the more extensive treatment required for their isolation may have caused a substantial loss of calcium. Addition of ATP to the suspension medium after isolation is not able to increase the calcium level. Hence, we prefer to use frog rods for studies of the light effect on the calcium content.

Contamination cannot explain the high calcium levels in our preparations. The minor mitochondrial contamination of the frog outer segment preparations could not account for more than a tiny fraction of the calcium content. In agreement with this we shall later see that oligomycin does not affect accumulation of calcium by outer segments. Contamination with pigment epithelium material could also be a source of error in view of the high calcium content in this tissue recently observed by Hess (1975). However, the slight contamination with melanin granules in our preparations cannot be responsible either, since increasing the number of filtration steps during isolation decreases the melanin content but not the calcium/rhodopsin ratio. Binding of "non-outer segment" calcium to the outer segment membranes during isolation is also unlikely, since treatment of the outer segment preparation with EDTA-containing Ringer solution does not lower the calcium level (Table 3.1). Incubation of the isolated frog rods in Ringer solution containing 5 x 10^{-5}M of the divalent cation ionophore A23187 for 30 min. lowers the calcium level by about 50%, which may fit in with the ionophore effects reported by Hagins and Yoshikami (1974). Hence, it seems reasonable to assume that rod outer segments do indeed contain a large amount of calcium sequestered in their interior. The fact that isolation in ATP-free medium lowers the calcium level by about 35% (Table 3.1) suggests the presence of an energy-dependent calcium uptake mechanism.

COMPARTMENTATION OF CALCIUM IN ROD OUTER SEGMENTS

We have investigated the existence of separate calcium pools in outer segments by determining the calcium content before and after osmotic lysis (Hendriks et al, 1974). Lysis is induced by adding 4 vol. water (or 10 mM EDTA) to the suspension, followed by vigorous shaking on a Vortex mixer for 10 sec. Light microscopy indicates that this procedure causes complete disruption of the typical outer segment structure and that only small fragments (max. 5μ) remain visible. Calcium determinations after centrifugation show that a substantial part of the calcium is solubilized after lysis by dilution with water (Table 3.2). The effect is larger for a preparation suspended previously in ATP-free Ringer solution. Lysis by dilution with 10 mM EDTA (or EGTA) removes nearly all calcium from the sediment.

Lysis of isolated cattle rod outer segments by the addition of 4 vols. H_2O reduces the sedimentable calcium fraction to 45% (S.E.: 2.2, 3 expts.). Magnesium in frog outer segments is also distributed over the two fractions. Lysis by the addition of 4 vols. H_2O gives a sedimentable fraction of 18% (S.E.: 0.6, 4 detns.), suggesting that the intra- to extrasaccular ratio is lower for this ionic species than for calcium.

These observations indicate that a particulate and a soluble calcium (and magnesium) fraction can be distinguished by the lysis method. The particulate calcium fraction coincides with the rhodopsin-containing sediment. Since the rod sacs are the only intracellular compartments in the outer segment, it is reasonable to assume that the particulate calcium fraction represents calcium which is present inside surviving intact rod sacs and/or which is bound to rod sac membranes. The effects of omission of ATP and of lysis in 10 mM EDTA (or EGTA) may suggest that part of the calcium is inside the rod sacs and part is bound to the rod sac membrane. We wish to emphasize, however, that

Table 3.2. Calcium distribution in intact and lysed frog rod outer segments

Suspension medium	Ringer + ATP	Ringer - ATP	Ringer + 10 mM EDTA
Lysis by 4 vols.:	H_2O	H_2O	10 mM EDTA
Before lysis	75 ± 4.7 (13)	59 ± 5.7 (9)	69 ± 0.8 (3)
After lysis	46 ± 2.0 (27)	29 ± 3.4 (4)	4.2 ± 2.2 (3)

Isolated rod outer segments are washed twice with the indicated Ringer-type solution, the sediment is resuspended and divided into different aliquots. After lysis by addition of 4 vols. water of 10 mM EDTA. All preparations are centrifuged and calcium is determined in sediments and supernatants. Results are expressed as the percentage of total calcium present in the sediment with standard error of the mean and in parentheses the number of experiments (each in triplicate).

the observed sedimentable/soluble calcium ratios do not represent the in vivo ratio of intra- to extrasaccular calcium, which is undoubtedly much higher. An upper limit of 5×10^{-6}M for the extrasaccular calcium concentration has been deduced from electrophysiological experiments in the presence of the ionophore X537A by Hagins and Yoshikami (1974), suggesting an in vivo ratio of over 10,000.

LIGHT-INDUCED SHIFTS IN CALCIUM DISTRIBUTION

We have first determined the effect of light on the total calcium content of frog outer segments (Hendriks et al, 1974). Rod outer segments suspended in a Ringer solution are illuminated immediately after sampling. Illumination is either by one or more flashes from a Rollei Strobofix E 60 flash lamp behind a Schott-Jena OG 2 filter (the first flash causing 50% bleaching of the rhodopsin present), or by a 100 W tungsten lamp for 5 min. behind 3 mm GG 3 and OG 2 filters (yielding nearly 85% bleaching). They are then immediately centrifuged, and calcium is determined both in the sediment and supernatant.

Illumination by either method causes no significant change in the percentage of total calcium remaining in the sediment, as compared to non-illuminated controls (Table 3.3). The presence or absence of 3 mM ATP or 10 mM EDTA does not make any difference in the results. Our conclusion is that the overall calcium content of intact isolated rod outer segments does not change upon illumination. This is not surprising, even if there would be a light-induced release of calcium from the rod sacs, since the permeability of the outer membrane to calcium should be very low, considering that washing intact outer segments twice does not significantly lower their calcium content.

Table 3.3. Effect of illumination on calcium content of intact frog rod outer segments

Medium	Outer segment sediment		Ratio light/dark	No. of expts.	No. of detns.	P-value *
	dark	light				
	%	%				
Ringer + 3 mM ATP	68.3	72.4	1.06	10	50	0.13
Ringer + ATP + 10 mM EDTA	67.9	67.7	1.00	2	12	0.23
Ringer - ATP	56.1	57.9	1.03	5	30	0.21

Isolated rod outer segments are washed twice in the indicated medium, and the sediment is resuspended and divided into 4-6 aliquots. Half of the aliquots are kept in darkness, the others are illuminated. After centrifugation calcium is determined in sediments and supernatants. Results are expressed as percent of total calcium present in the sediment.

*Determined by two-way analysis of variance.

Combining lysis and illumination, we have determined the effect of illumination on the distribution of calcium between the sedimentable and soluble fractions. When intact, frog rod outer segments are flash illuminated and then lysed by addition of 4 vols. H_2O, a significant loss of calcium into the supernatant occurs, as compared to non-illuminated controls (Table 3.4, upper row). This means that illumination causes a shift of calcium from the sedimentable to the soluble fraction, suggesting that in the intact rod cell light shifts calcium from the rod sacs to the extrasaccular space.

Table 3.4. Light-induced loss of particulate calcium of frog rod outer segments

Outer segment treatment	Sedimentable fraction Dark	Light	Percent calcium lost by illumination	No. of expts.	No. of detns.	P-value *
Lysis after illumination	42.8	36.0	16	4	28	0.01
Lysis before illumination	41.5	39.0	6	3	22	0.85
Lysis, centrifugation, resuspension in ATP-Ringer, illumination	38.9	28.7	26	5	31	0.001

Isolated frog rod outer segments are washed twice with ATP-containing Ringer solution and centrifuged, the sediment is resuspended in the same solution and divided into aliquots. These are treated as indicated in the first column. Lysis is by addition of 4 vols. H_2O. Illumination is by flashing so as to give maximal bleaching (85%). After centrifugation calcium is determined in sediment and supernatant. Results are expressed as the percentage of calcium present in the sediment, and also as the relative loss of calcium upon illumination.

*Determined by two-way analysis of variance.

By reversing the sequence, i.e. illuminating after lysis, we have tried to establish whether the calcium content of the sedimentable fraction after disruption of the outer segment is still sensitive to light. Rod outer segments are lysed in darkness, the preparation is immediately illuminated and centrifuged. No significant effect of light is seen (Table 3.4, second row). However, when the lysed preparation is first centrifuged and the sediment resuspended in isotonic Ringer solution, subsequent illumination gives a significant loss of sedimentable calcium again (Table 3.4, third row). This suggests that the mechanism by which particulate calcium is released upon illumination remains intact upon lysis. The need to resuspend the lysed material first in isotonic Ringer solution suggests that either the low ionic concentrations (Na^+, K^+, Mg^{2+}) in the 5x diluted Ringer solution or the relatively high calcium concentration in the medium after lysis (approx. 10^{-5}M) inhibits the light-sensitive calcium release mechanism.

Light has no effect on the magnesium distribution. Illumination of the lysed rod outer segments, after resuspension in isotonic magnesium-free Ringer solution (required for accuracy of the magnesium determination), gives a sedimentable fraction of 18.5% (S.E. 0.6, 4 detns.), compared to 18.1% (S.E. 0.6, 4 detns.) without illumination. The relative loss of sedimentable calcium upon illumination is under these circumstances 9.2% (S.E. 0.2, 4 paired detns.). Although this calcium loss is only about half of that in a magnesium-containing Ringer solution, the effect is still significant. This finding indicates that the light-induced calcium release is specific for this bivalent ion. The smaller light effect in the magnesium-free medium may indicate that magnesium plays a role in the release mechanism.

In another series of experiments we have begun to investigate the relation between the percentage bleaching of rhodopsin and the loss of calcium from lysed frog outer segment material (Table 3.5). The outer segments are lysed again by addition of 4 vols. H_2O, centrifuged, resuspended in ATP containing Ringer solution, and flash illuminated at increasing distance between sample and flash apparatus. Decreasing the light intensity so as to bleach only 15% of the rhodopsin does not lower the loss of calcium from the sedimentable fraction. One would, of course, want to know at what bleaching percentage the relative calcium loss would begin to decrease. Unfortunately, recently imposed legal restrictions on the use of frogs for experimental purposes in the Netherlands have made it impossible for us to extend these experiments to still lower bleaching levels. The few frogs available since then have been of different varieties and sources, and have not given consistent results. However, Szuts and Cone (1974) report in an abstract finding a 50% release at 1%

Table 3.5. Light-induced loss of particulate calcium of frog rod outer segments as a function of percent rhodopsin bleached

Percent rhodopsin bleached	Percent particulate calcium lost
85	24 ± 1.2 (5)
40	19 (1)
15	27 ± 3.9 (5)

Isolated frog rod outer segment are washed twice with ATP-containing Ringer solution and centrifuged, the sediment is resuspended in the same evolution and divided into aliquots. These are lysed by addition of 4 vols. water, centrifuged, resuspended in ATP-Ringer solution, and illuminated at the required distances from the flash apparatus. After centrifugation calcium is determined in sediment and supernatant of both illuminated and non-illuminated samples. Results are expressed as the relative loss of sedimentable calcium upon illumination.

bleaching and in some cases even at 0.01% bleaching. Mason et al (1974) claim to have observed a fast light-induced ^{45}Ca release from preloaded frog rod outer segment preparations in the presence of EGTA, but fail to show control experiments in darkness with EGTA present. Weller et al (1975) report an increased ^{45}Ca efflux from preloaded bovine rod outer segment preparations, but here the effect appears to be substantial only after a relatively long time interval ($>$8 min.).

Since we have found that 12.4 moles calcium are present per mol rhodopsin in intact frog rods, a 27% loss of sedimentable calcium at 15% bleaching would imply a release of about 22 calcium ions per molecule of rhodopsin bleached. This figure, which is probably a lower limit for the value at single photon absorption, falls within the range of 3-300 calcium ions per photon estimated by Yoshikami and Hagins (1973) to reduce the dark current by the 3% observed for a single absorbed photon.

PERMEABILITY OF PHOSPHOLIPID BILAYERS FOR CALCIUM AND SODIUM IONS

Both the light-induced release of calcium ions from rod sacs and the light-regulated entry of sodium ions across the outer membrane would appear to involve passive movements of these ions through the relevant biomembranes. In the hope of learning more about these processes we have studied the movement of calcium and sodium through artificial phospholipid bilayers (Hyono et al, 1975; Hendriks, 1975).

We have made use of liposomes, multi-layered vesicles of varying lipid composition, containing a radioisotope of the ion to be studied (see e.g.: Bangham, 1968). Briefly, the technique is as follows. The lipid or lipid mixture (40 mg) is deposited as a thin film on the inside of a flask by rotating evaporation of the organic solvent. A buffered salt solution (4 ml) containing the ion (and its radioisotope) to be tested is added. The mixture is shaken vigorously for 30 min. in a nitrogen atmosphere, and then left for 2 h. at room temperature. Radioactive ions which have not been trapped in the liposomes are removed by gel filtration over a Sephadex G-50 column. Samples of 1 ml of the resulting liposome suspension are placed in small dialysis bags. The closed bags are placed in test tubes containing 10-12 ml of the isotope-free salt solution. The stoppered test tubes are attached to a vertically rotating disk (1 rev./min.). Over a 2-3 h. period samples of the outer solution are withdrawn for radioactive counting at 20-min. intervals. At the end of the experiment the radioactivity remaining inside the dialysis bag is also counted.

The liposomes have been prepared from phosphatidylcholine, phosphatidylserine, a mixture of the two, a lipid extract of whole cattle retina, and one of cattle rod outer segments. The capture of ^{22}Na and ^{45}Ca in the various types of liposomes is shown in Table 3.6. Capture of calcium is always higher than that of sodium. Liposomes made of rod outer segment lipids give less capture for either ion than those made of retinal lipids. Parallel relationships exist for the efflux rates: the efflux rate for calcium is always lower than that for sodium (Fig. 3.2), while the efflux rates for both ions are much higher in rod outer segment lipid liposomes than in retinal lipid liposomes.

Table 3.6. Capture of radioactive ions by various types of liposomes

Liposomes composition	^{22}Na	^{45}Ca
	%	%
Phosphatidylcholine	0.6	1
Phosphatidylcholine-phosphatidylserine, 4:1	1.2	4
Retinal lipids	5.2	12.8
Rod outer segment lipids	0.7	1.8

Liposome preparation is described in the text. Results are expressed as percent of total radioactivity eluted from the Sephadex G-50 column, present in the liposomal fraction.

The high permeability of the outer segment lipid liposomes requires an explanation. It cannot be the phospholipid composition, since that is about the same as that for the whole retina (Daemen, 1973). However, the fatty acid composition of these two lipid fractions is quite different (Table 3.7). The outer segment lipids have 2x as much docosahexaenic (C 22:6) acid and their average number of double bonds per fatty acid molecule is 1.5 x as high. Simultaneously the outer segment lipids contain only 1/3 as much cholesterol as the retinal lipids. These two differences could very well explain the much higher permeability of the outer segment lipid liposomes (cf. De Gier et al, 1968).

In view of the alleged role of calcium ions in lowering the sodium permeability of the outer membrane of the rod outer segment, it was interesting to investigate whether such an effect could be demonstrated in the liposomes. In 16 expts. with various types of liposomes addition of 5 mM Ca^{2+} to the dialysis medium causes an average decrease of 20% ($P < 0.001$) in the ^{22}Na efflux rate during the first 30 minutes (Hendriks, 1975). It would be interesting to observe whether incorporation of protein, esp. rhodopsin, in rod outer segment lipid liposomes would further increase the calcium sensitivity of the

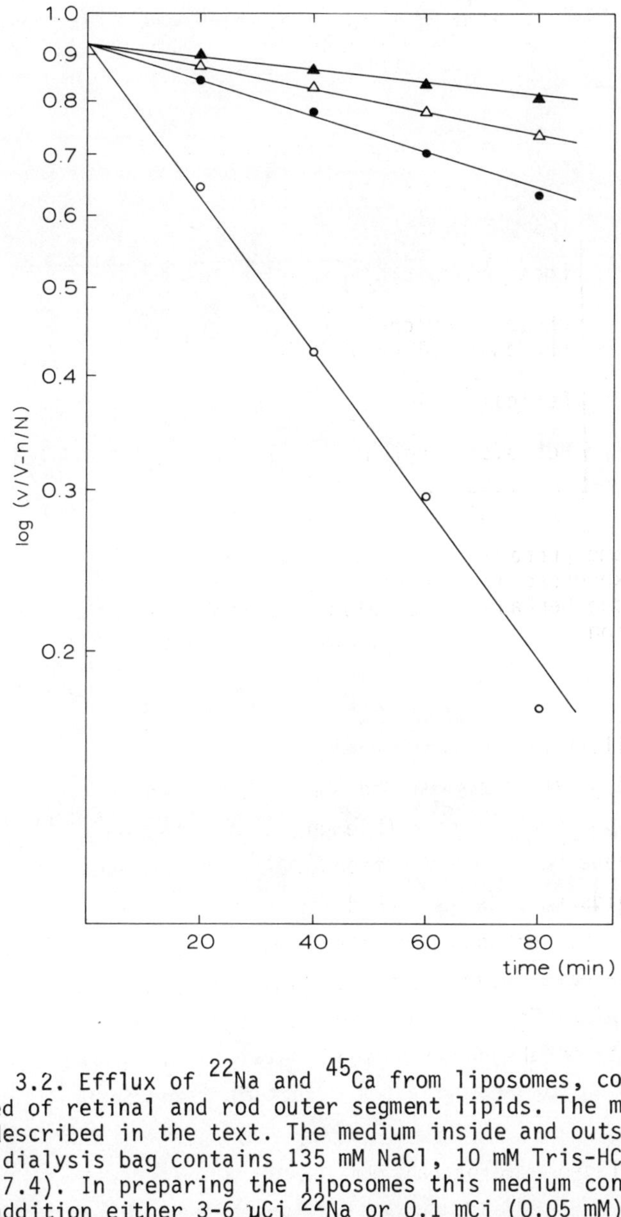

Fig. 3.2. Efflux of ^{22}Na and ^{45}Ca from liposomes, composed of retinal and rod outer segment lipids. The method is described in the text. The medium inside and outside the dialysis bag contains 135 mM NaCl, 10 mM Tris-HCl (pH 7.4). In preparing the liposomes this medium contains in addition either 3-6 µCi ^{22}Na or 0.1 mCi (0.05 mM) ^{45}Ca. Efflux rates are plotted as log (v/V - n/N) vs. time, where v is the fluid volume outside the dialysis bag, V the fluid volume inside and outside the dialysis bag, n is the number of counts outside the dialysis bag, N is the total number of counts. Theoretically, these should be straight lines (Hyono et al, 1975). The open symbols refer to ^{22}Na, the closed symbols to ^{45}Ca; triangles indicate retinal lipid liposomes, circles indicate rod outer segment lipid liposomes.

Table 3.7. Fatty acid composition and cholesterol content of lipids of whole cattle retina and cattle rod outer segments

Fatty acid (nr. of C atoms: nr. of double bonds)	Whole retina (2 prepns.)	Rod outer segments (3 prepns.)
16:0	20.2 ± 0.5	13.0 ± 0.9
16:1	1.0	0.4
18:0	19.9 ± 0.9	19.3 ± 0.2
18:1	10.7 ± 0.2	3.2 ± 0.3
18:2	1.4	0.7 ± 0.1
20:4	9.7 ± 0.7	5.4 ± 0.7
22:4/22:5	7.4 ± 2.2	8.2 ± 3.4
22:6	24.1 ± 3.5	48.2 ± 4.4
undet'd	5.6	1.6
cholesterol content	13.4 ± 0.2	4.3 ± 0.6

The major fatty acids are expressed as percentage of the total fatty acid content. Analysis by gas-liquid chromatography was kindly performed by Dr. R.M. Broekhuyse as previously described by him (Broekhuyse, 1972). Cholesterol was determined by the Liebermann-Burchard method (Hendriks, 1975).

sodium permeability. In such rhodopsin-containing liposomes another obvious experiment would be to determine the effect of light on their calcium permeability.

Calculation of the partition of calcium ions between liposomes and medium shows that a capture of 1% represents equal distribution. The higher figures for retinal lipid and outer segment lipid liposomes in Table 3.6 indicate considerable binding of calcium ions to the lipid bilayer. Utilization of the partition coefficient for the calculation of the free energy gives a value far too low for direct chemical binding; hence the calcium must be loosely and exchangeably bound to the polar head groups of the phospholipids (Hyono et al, 1975). This would also explain why the addition of a calcium ionophore like A23187 can increase the calcium efflux very greatly (100 x at 3 x 10^{-8}M A23187) in these experiments.

CALCIUM BINDING BY ROD OUTER SEGMENT MEMBRANES

For the remaining part of this chapter we shall address ourselves to the question of how the rod sacs accumulate and store the large amounts of calcium they appear to contain. There are two previously mentioned possibilities: binding to the rod sac membrane or accumulation across this membrane into the interior space of the rod sac. If the latter process operates, then passive binding of the ion to the membrane might have to precede active translocation across the membrane.

Therefore, we have examined passive binding of calcium to rod outer segments by means of the equilibrium dialysis technique (Hendriks, 1975). Other investigators have reported evidence for binding of calcium to rod sac membranes (Bownds et al, 1971; Neufeld et al, 1972; Mason et al, 1974; Hemminki, 1975), but their conditions and techniques do not allow a clear distinction between passive binding and active translocation.

Cattle rod outer segments are isolated according to a modification of the method of De Grip et al (1972): the final washing is in 15 mM EDTA (instead of H_2O) in order to remove calcium. The outer segments are suspended in a buffered salt solution (e.g. 100 mM NaCl, 20 mM Tris-HCl, pH 7.4), and 5-ml aliquots are placed in dialysis bags. The bags are closed, and placed in test tubes containing 10 ml of the same solution, to which 0.7 µCi ^{45}Ca and varying amounts of ^{40}Ca (10^{-5} to 5 x 10^{-3}M) are added. The stoppered tubes are attached to a vertically rotating disk (1 rev./min.). After dialysis for 40 h. at 4^{0}C, 500-µl samples are withdrawn from the solutions inside and outside the dialysis bag for radioactive counting. Recovery of ^{45}Ca is always better than 90%, usually between 95 and 100%. Percent bound ^{45}Ca is calculated from the excess of isotope inside the bags. After 40 h. dialysis equilibrium has been reached. Donnan equilibria do not play a detectable role.

The amounts of calcium bound in various media (calcium concentration always 10^{-5}M) is shown in Table 3.8. The largest amount of calcium bound is observed

Table 3.8. Calcium binding by cattle rod outer segment membranes: effect of medium

Medium	Binding (nmol calcium/mg protein)
20 mM Tris-HCl	8.2 ± 0.80 (2)
+ 100 mM NaCl	1.45 ± 0.17 (7)
+ 100 mM NaCl + 5 mM $MgCl_2$	0.64 ± 0.14 (4)
+ 100 mM KCl	1.10
+ 100 mM KCl + 5 mM $MgCl_2$	0.57

The procedure is described in the text. The calcium concentration is 10^{-5}M in all experiments. Experiments performed in dim red light.

in 20 mM Tris-HCl (pH 7.4), and is equivalent to 0.7 mol calcium per mol rhodopsin. Addition of 100 mM NaCl or KCl lowers this substantially, and addition of 5 mM $MgCl_2$ further decreases the amount of calcium bound. However, the fact that there is still significant binding of calcium at a sodium (or potassium) to calcium ratio of 10,000 and at a magnesium to calcium ratio of 500 indicates that the binding sites are rather specific for calcium. An important observation is that storage of the suspension overnight at 4°C or frozen at -70°C does not change the calcium binding capacity, neither does lyophilization of the material before equilibrium dialysis. Furthermore, addition of the calcium ionophore A23187 (10^{-7} - 10^{-5}M) does not decrease the amount of bound calcium (Table 3.9). This shows clearly that we are determining passive binding of calcium to membranes only and not active translocation.

Binding increases very markedly with increasing calcium concentration in the external medium (Fig. 3.3). Over the concentration range 10^{-5} to 5 x 10^{-3}M binding rises from 1 to 134 nmol calcium per mg protein, or 0.06 to 8.1 mol calcium per mol rhodopsin. These data have been transformed into a Scatchard

Table 3.9. Calcium binding by cattle rod outer segment membranes: effect of ionophore A23187

Calcium concentration (M)	ionophore concentration (M)			
	0	10^{-7}	10^{-6}	10^{-5}
10^{-5}	1.5 ± 0.17	1.5 ± 0.02	1.6 ± 0.05	2.2 ± 0.23
10^{-3}	53 ± 0.3	53 ± 11.1	55 ± 3.7	67 ± 4.5

The procedure is described in the text. Medium composition is 100 mM NaCl + 20 mM Tris-HCl (pH 7.4). Ionophore is added to the dialysis medium. Results, expressed as nmol calcium bound per mg. protein, are averages of two experiments (± half the range).

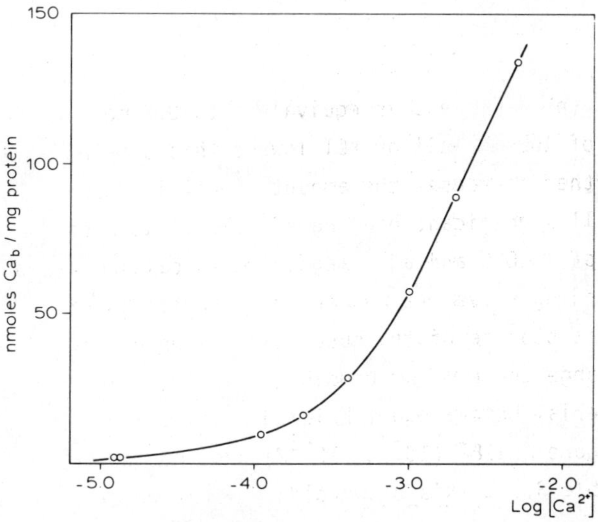

Fig. 3.3. Concentration dependence of calcium binding by cattle rod outer segments. Medium composition: 100 mM NaCl, 20 mM Tris-HCl (pH 7.4). The calcium concentration in the dialysis medium is varied from 10^{-5} to 5×10^{-3}M. Experiments performed in dim red light.

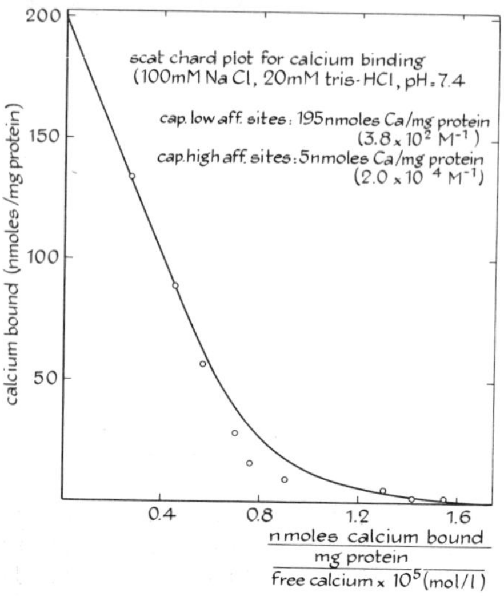

Fig. 3.4. Scatchard plot for calcium binding by cattle rod outer segment membranes. The data of Fig. 3.3 have been converted (open circles). The best fitting theoretical curve for a total binding capacity of 200 nmol calcium per mg membrane protein has been computed and is shown.

plot (Fig. 3.4), which permits us to determine the relative binding affinities and the binding capacities of the various binding sites. Extrapolation to infinitely high calcium concentration shows that the maximal binding capacity is 200 nmol/mg protein (12 mol/mol rhodopsin). The best fitting theoretical curve at this total binding capacity has been computed. This curve is biphasic, indicating that there are two types of binding sites with different binding affinities. The low-affinity sites have a capacity of about 195 nmol/mg protein and an affinity of $3.8 \times 10^2 M^{-1}$; for the high-affinity sites these numbers are approx. 5 nmol/mg protein and $2.0 \times 10^4 M^{-1}$. Hemminki (1975) also concludes that there are two types of binding sites. He finds capacities of 210 and 25 nmol/mg protein, and affinity constants of 86 M^{-1} and $2.5 \times 10^3 M^{-1}$, respectively. So his affinity constants are only about 1/8 - 1/4 of those found by us. This may be due to his use of the Millipore filtration technique, which may lead to a loss of bound calcium and hence to apparently lower affinities.

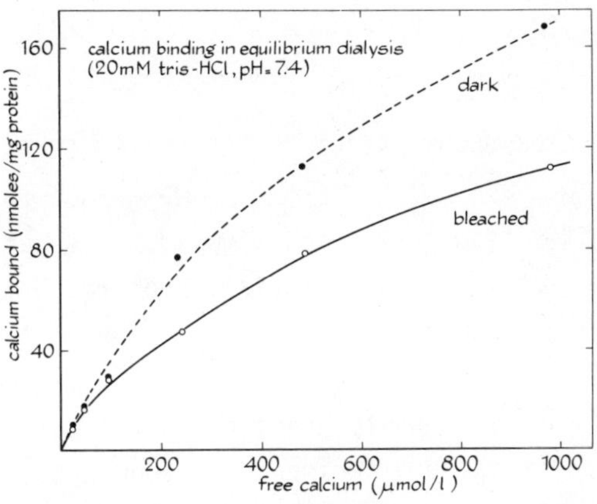

Fig. 3.5. Effect of light on calcium binding by cattle rod outer segments. Medium composition: 20 mM Tris-HCl (pH 7.4). The calcium concentration in the dialysis medium has been varied from 2 x 10^{-5} to 10^{-3}M. Experiments performed in dim red light (closed circles) or light (open circles). At calcium levels equal to or below 5 x 10^{-5}M no light effect is observed, while at higher calcium levels the percentage decreases by a steady 34%.

There is some effect of light on calcium binding (Fig. 3.5), but only at calcium levels above 5 x 10^{-5}M. For calcium levels between 10^{-4} to 10^{-3}M light reduces binding by one third. These findings are in agreement with those of Hemminki (1975), and with those of Neufeld et al (1972), who find no effect of light but use calcium concentrations of max. 10^{-5}M. It appears from this concentration dependence that light does not affect the high-affinity sites, but only the low-affinity sites. The number of the latter sites (12 per rhodopsin molecule) suggests that they represent acid groups of phospholipids in the rod sac membrane. The relatively few (0.3 per rhodopsin molecule) high-affinity sites may be associated with an active calcium translocation system, as is assumed for sarcoplasmic reticulum (Chevallier and Butow, 1971) and for mitochondria (Reynafarje and Lehninger, 1969). If the estimate of the extra-saccular calcium concentration ($<$2 x 10^{-6}M) by Hagins and Yoshikami (1974) is correct, then less than 0.3 mol calcium per mol rhodopsin would be passively bound to the outside of the rod sac membranes. Since we find frog and cattle roud outer segments to contain 12.4 and 2.5 mol calcium per mol rhodopsin, this suggests that the major part of this calcium must be accumulated in another way, viz. by translocation into the rod sacs. The latter process will now be considered.

CALCIUM ACCUMULATION IN ROD OUTER SEGMENTS

For the study of active transport of calcium into rod outer segments it is essential to have intact and fresh material. Frog rod outer segments would have been preferable, but current legal restriction of the use of frogs in the Netherlands has made this difficult. Hence, cattle rod outer segments, freshly isolated by sucrose density gradient centrifugation (De Grip et al, 1972), have been used in these experiments. Although the high purity of this preparation is an advantage, it is more difficult to obtain these outer segments in an intact state. This is noticeable in the difficulty to obtain high, reproducible calcium/rhodopsin ratio's. Lowering the osmolarity of the gradient fluid by replacing part of the sucrose by Ficoll (13% Ficoll + 25% sucrose instead of 40% sucrose) appears to improve the calcium accumulation, possibly because there is less osmotic shrinkage of the rod sacs in this medium. Through the addition of 1 mM EGTA to the buffer solution, in which the outer segments are isolated, maximal depletion of endogenous calcium (to less than 0.1 mol/mol rhodopsin) is archieved. This ensures proportionality between ^{45}Ca and total calcium, so that the isotope distribution gives a reliable estimate of the total calcium distribution. Depending on the calcium concentration, rod/medium gradients of 10-20 can be achieved in this way.

The freshly isolated outer segments are incubated for 45 min. at 25°C in a salt solution, normally containing 100 mM KCl, 2 mM $MgCl_2$, 1 mM ATP, 50 µM $CaCl_2$, 1 µCi/ml ^{45}Ca, 20 mM Tris-HCl (pH 7.4). At various time intervals 200 µl aliquots of the suspension are pipetted into 2.5 ml of the same salt solution, lacking ^{45}Ca and containing in addition 0.1 mM EGTA (to remove adhering calcium), on a borosilicate glass fiber filter. After adding an additional 2.5 ml salt solution, the mixture is immediately filtered by suction. The filtration procedure takes 4-6 sec. Radioactive counting of the material on the filter and determination of the rhodopsin content permits calculation of the calcium/rhodopsin ratio. Ratio's of 1-6, depending on the calcium concentration in the incubation medium, are obtained.

The effects of ATP and of the major cation are shown in Fig. 3.6. The accumu-

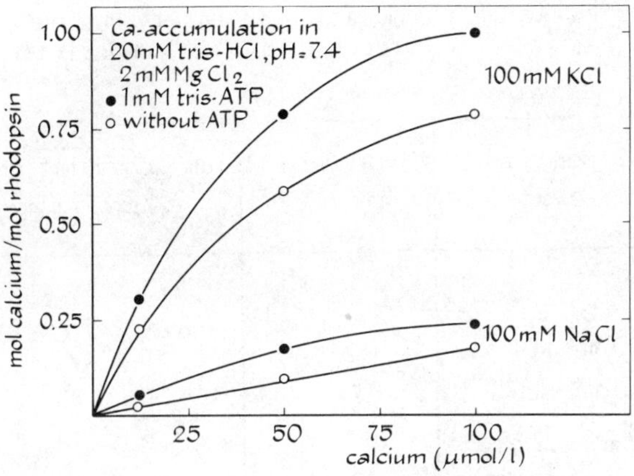

Fig. 3.6. Calcium accumulation in cattle rod outer segments. Uptake media contain: 100 mM KCl or NaCl, 2 mM $MgCl_2$, 0 or 1 mM ATP, 13,50 or 100 μm $CaCl_2$, 1 μCi ^{45}Ca, 20 mM Tris-HCl (pH 7.4). The procedure is described in the text. Closed circles: 1 mM ATP, open circles: 0 mM ATP.

lation is much higher in the presence of 100 mM KCl than in that of 100 mM NaCl. The presence of 1 mM ATP increases the accumulation by about 25%. The effects of further variations in the medium are shown in Table 3.10. Only isosmotic replacement of KCl by sucrose gives somewhat higher accumulation. In further experiments the KCl medium has been routinely used.

There are various arguments favoring the assumption that we are here observing an uptake across a membrane (most likely the rod sac membrane), and not a binding process as in the equilibrium dialysis experiments:

1. freezing or lyophilization of the outer segments prior to incubation greatly reduces or even abolishes the accumulation of ^{45}Ca.
2. there is a (partial) dependence on ATP, the optimal concentration range being 0.2 - 1.0 mM.
3. the accumulation greatly depends on the major cation present in the medium, which is not the case in the equilibrium dialysis experiments.
4. addition of the calcium ionophore A23187 (10^{-5}M) to the medium after accumulation rapidly and largely abolishes the ^{45}Ca gradient in the outer segments (Fig. 3.7).

The question that immediately arises is: does this accumulation process repre-

Table 3.10. Calcium accumulation in cattle rod outer segments: effects of medium composition

Medium	Relative calcium accumulation - ATP	+ ATP (1 mM)
	%	%
100 mM KCl	= 100	= 100
100 mM NaCl	17	23
100 mM Tris	100	78
100 mM sucrose	92	89
200 mM sucrose	167	128

The medium contains in addition: 20 mM Tris-HCl (pH 7.4). 2 mM $MgCl_2$, 50 μM $CaCl_2$, 1 μCi/ml ^{45}Ca.
The procedure is as described in the text.

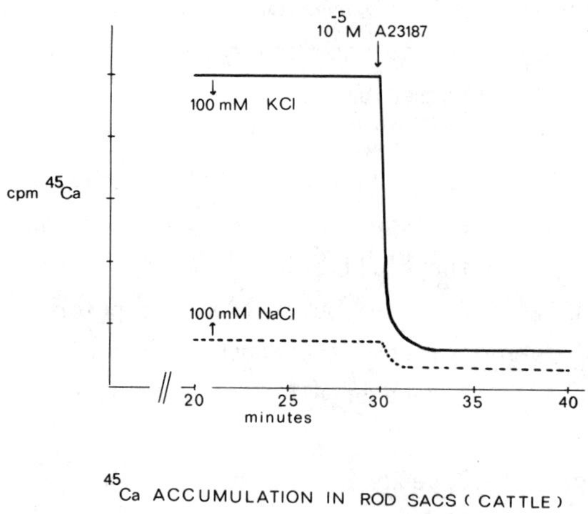

Fig. 3.7. Abolishing of calcium gradient in cattle rod outer segments by calcium ionophore A23187 (10^{-5}M). The further procedure is described in the text.

sent active transport of calcium into the rod sacs?

Active transport of calcium has been extensively studied in sarcoplasmic reticulum (Hasselbach, 1974), mitochondria (Lehninger et al, 1967) and erythrocytes (Schatzmann and Rossi, 1971). In an attempt to compare the rod outer segment mechanism with that of these other systems, the effects of substances known to inhibit calcium transport in one or more of the latter have been tested (Table 3.11). Oligomycin, ruthenium red and lanthanum ion, which inhibit calcium accumulation in mitochondria (Reed and Bygrave, 1974), have no inhibitory effect; in the case of lanthanum there is even some stimulation. Apparently, the transport mechanism in outer segments is rather different from that in these other systems. The absence of an inhibitory effect of ouabain suggests that calcium transport in outer segments is not coupled to the ouabain-sensitive sodium pump.

Table 3.11. Calcium accumulation is cattle rod outer segments: effects of various inhibitors

Substance added	Relative calcium accumulation	
	- ATP	+ ATP (1 mM)
	%	%
none	= 100	= 100
oligomycin, 5 µg/ml	95	97
ruthenium red, 0.1 mM	97	102
$LaCl_3$, 0.04 mM	106	135
ouabain, 0.1 mM	102	103

The medium contains in addition: 100 mM KCl, 2 mM $MgCl_2$, 50 µM $CaCl_2$, 1 µCi/ml ^{45}Ca, 20 mM Tris-HCl (pH 7.4). The procedure is as described in the text.

In view of these findings it is perhaps not surprising that the search for a transport ATPase has not yet yielded clear results. In cattle rod outer segments an ATPase activity has been demonstrated (Hendriks, 1975), which is sti-

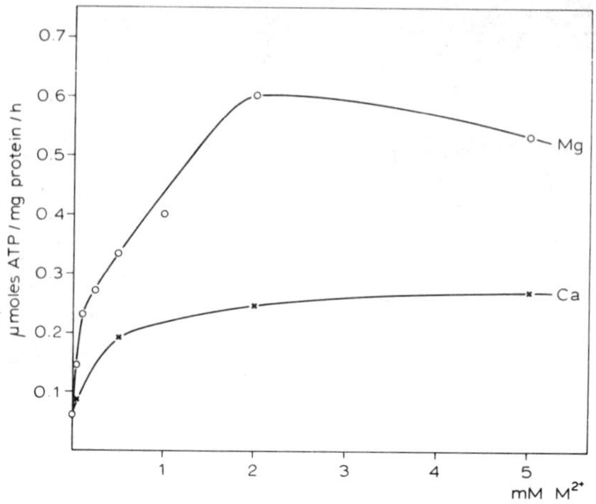

Fig. 3.8. Effects of calcium and magnesium on ATPase activity in cattle rod outer segments. Lyophilized outer segments, isolated by density gradient centrifugation, are reconstituted with water, and the bivalent cation-activated ATPase activity is determined in a medium containing in addition to calcium or magnesium: 2 mM Tris-ATP and 100 mM Tris HCl (pH 7.5). After incubation for 60 min. at 37°C inorganic phosphate is measured as described by Bonting (1970, p. 263).

mulated by either magnesium or calcium (Fig. 3.8). Lineweaver-Burke plots, calculated from the values shown in Fig. 3.8 and corrected for the activity without bivalent cation, do not yield straight lines. Hence, it is impossible to measure reliable K_m values. Approximate values are 5×10^{-4}M and 4×10^{-5}M for magnesium and calcium, respectively. When calcium (10^{-5} - 10^{-2}M) is added to a medium containing 2 mM $MgCl_2$, 2 mM Tris-ATP, 100 mM Tris-HCl (pH 7.5), a decrease rather than stimulation of the ATPase activity is noticed (Fig. 3.9). In the presence of 5 mM calcium + 2 mM magnesium the activity is about the same as that with 5 mM calcium alone. Addition of 55 mM NaCl, 5 mM KCl, 0.1 mM EGTA and 0.1 mM ouabain does not alter these results. Thus, we have so far only found a (Ca or Mg)- activated ATPase activity, but not a (Ca + Mg)-activated ATPase activity as occurs in sarcoplasmic reticulum and erythrocytes. In the absence of a common inhibitor for this enzyme activity and the calcium accumulation process in outer segments, it is impossible to know whether this enzyme activity has any relation to a calcium transport system.

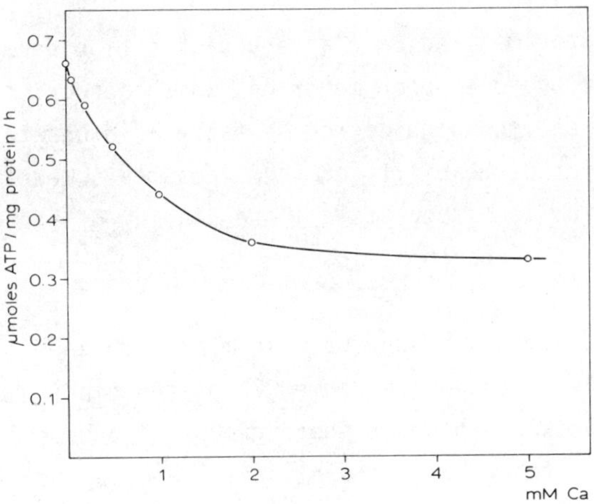

Fig. 3.9. Effect of calcium on the magnesium-activated ATPase activity in cattle rod outer segments. Calcium (10^{-6} - 10^{-2}M) is added to a medium containing: 2 mM $MgCl_2$, 2 mM Tris-ATP, 100 mM Tris-HCl (pH 7.5). ATPase activity is measured as described in the legend of Fig. 3.8.

CONCLUDING REMARKS

The hypothesis of Hagins that calcium ions would play a role as an intracellular transmitter in photoreceptor excitation has been tested in various ways.

Frog and cattle rod outer segments have a remarkably high calcium content, when they are isolated rapidly and with certain precautions (presence of ATP, avoiding damage). Osmotic lysis of isolated frog rod outer segments indicates that the calcium is mainly located in the rhodopsin-containing compartment, presumably the rod sacs.

Illumination releases no calcium from intact outer segments, but lysis before or after illumination allows establishing a light-induced release of calcium, but not of magnesium, from the sedimentable calcium pool. The amount of calcium released per bleached rhodopsin molecule, if extrapolation to the single photon level is valid, would satisfy the conditions formulated by Hagins from his electrophysiological studies.

Efflux studies on liposomes indicate a very high cation permeability of the lipid bilayer in the photoreceptor membrane, which appears to be due to the low cholesterol content and high degree of fatty acid unsaturation. Calcium ions reduce the sodium permeability of the liposomes somewhat. The high capture value for calcium ions suggests a loose binding of these ions to the polar head groups of the phospholipids.

Passive binding of calcium ions on outer segment membranes is demonstrated by the equilibrium dialysis technique. Some 97% of the binding sites have a low affinity and may represent the polar head groups of phospholipids. Three percent of the binding sites have a high affinity, and may be associated with an active calcium translocation system. Illumination decreases low-affinity binding by one third, but not the high-affinity binding. At the presumed low cytoplasmic calcium concentration the low-affinity sites would hardly be occupied, which would imply that passive binding cannot explain the high calcium content of the outer segments.

Uptake studies with ^{45}Ca indicate the existence of a calcium translocation system. Its properties differ from those of the sarcoplasmic reticulum, mitochondrial and erythrocyte translocation systems. A bivalent cation stimulated ATPase activity, which is present in the outer segment, does not display a synergistic effect for Ca^{2+} + Mg^{2+}. It is uncertain whether this ATPase activity is associated with the calcium translocation.

Some of the techniques, applied and evolved in this study, should be capable of providing further insight in the role of calcium in vision and of avoiding the many pitfalls endangering the investigator studying the biological functions of calcium ions.

ACKNOWLEDGEMENTS

The autors gratefully acknowledge the permission given by Dr. T. Hendriks and Mr. P. Schnetkamp for quoting from their unpublished results. They also acknowledge the advice and criticism of Mr. Schnetkamp in preparing this chapter. The research in their laboratory has been supported in part by the

Netherlands Foundation for Basic Research (ZWO) through the Netherlands Foundation for Chemical Research (SON).

REFERENCES

Baker P.F. (1972) Transport and metabolism of calcium ions in nerve. Progr. Biophys. Mol. Biol. 24, 177-223.

Bangham A.D. (1968) Membrane models with phospholipids. Progr. Biophys. Mol. Biol. 18, 29-95.

Bonting S.L. (1970) Sodium-potassium activated adenosinetriphosphatase and cation transport, in: Membranes and Ion Transport (Bittar E.E. ed.), Vol. I, pp. 257-363, Wiley-Interscience, New York.

Bownds D., Gordon-Walker A., Gaide-Huguenin A.C. and Robinson W. (1971) Characterization and analysis of frog photoreceptor membranes. J. Gen. Physiol. 58, 225-237.

Broekhuyse R.M. (1972) Lipids in tissues of the eye. VII Changes in concentration and composition of lipids in aging sclera. Biochim. Biophys. Acta 280, 637-645.

Chevallier J. and Butow R.A. (1971) Calcium binding to the sarcoplasmic reticulum of rabbit skeletal muscle. Biochemistry 10, 2733-2737.

Daemen F.J.M. (1973) Vertebrate rod outer segments. Biochim. Biophys. Acta 300, 255-288.

Gier J. de, Mandersloot J.G. and Deenen L.L.M. van (1968) Lipid composition and permeability of liposomes. Biochim. Biophys. Acta 150, 666-675.

Grip W.J. de, Daemen F.J.M. and Bonting S.L. (1972) Biochemical aspects of the visual process. XVIII. Enrichment of rhodopsin in rod outer segment preparations. Vision Res. 12, 1697-1707.

Hagins W.A., Penn R.D., Yoshikami S. (1970) Dark current and photocurrent in retinal rods. Biophys. J. 10, 380-412.

Hagins W.A. (1972) The visual process: excitatory mechanism in the primary receptor cells. Ann. Rev. Biophys. Bioeng. 1. 131-158.

Hagins W.A. and Yoshikami S. (1974) Role for calcium in excitation of retinal rods and cones. Exp. Eye Res. 18, 299-305.

Hasselbach W. (1974) Sarcoplasmic membrane ATPases, in: The Enzymes (Boyer P.D. ed.), Vol. X, pp. 431-467, Acad. Press, New York.

Hemminki K. (1975) Light-induced decrease in calcium binding to isolated bovine photoreceptors. Vision Res. 15, 69-72.

Hendriks T., Pont J.J.H.H.M. de, Daemen F.J.M. and Bonting S.L. (1973) Biochemical aspects of the visual process. XXIV. Adenylate cyclase and rod photoreceptor membranes: a critical appraisal. Biochim. Biophys. Acta 330, 156-166.

Hendriks T., Daemen F.J.M. and Bonting S.L. (1974) Biochemical aspects of the visual process. XXV. Light-induced calcium movements in isolated frog rod outer segments. Biochim. Biophys. Acta 345, 468-473.

Hendriks T. (1975) The role of calcium and cyclic AMP in visual excitation. Ph.D. Thesis, Univ. of Nijmegen, Krips, Meppel

Hess H. (1975) The high calcium content of retinal pigmented epithelium. Exp. Eye Res. 21, oct. 15 issue, Current Contents.

Hyono A., Hendriks T., Daemen F.J.M. and Bonting S.L. (1975) Movement of calcium through artificial lipid membranes and the effects of ionophores. Biochim. Biophys. Acta 389, 34-46.

Korenbrot J.I. and Cone R.A. (1972) Dark ionic flux and the effects of light in isolated rod outer segments. J. Gen. Physiol. 60, 20-45.

Lehninger A.L., Carafoli E. and Rossi C.S. (1967) Energy-linked ion movements in mitochondrial systems. Advan. Enzymol. 29, 259-320.

Liebman P.A. (1962) In situ microspectrophotometric studies on the pigments of single retinal rods. Biophys. J. 2, 161-178.

Liebman P.A. (1974) Light-dependent calcium content of rod outer segment disc membranes. Invest. Ophthalmol. 13, 700-701.

Mason W.T., Fager R.S. and Abrahamson E.W. (1974) Ion fluxes in disk membranes of retinal rod outer segments. Nature 247, 562-563.

Neufeld A.H., Miller W.H. and Bitensky M.W. (1972) Calcium binding to retinal rod disk membranes. Biochim. Biophys. Acta 266, 67-71.

Reed K.C. and Bygrave F.L. (1974) Biochem. J. 140, 143-155.

Reynafarje B. and Lehninger A.L. (1969) High affinity and low affinity binding of calcium by rat liver mitochondria. J. Biol Chem. 244, 584-593.

Schatzmann H.J. and Rossi G.L. (1971) Calcium-magnesium activated membrane ATPases in human red cells and their possible relations to cation transport. Biochim. Biophys. Acta 241, 379-392.

Szuts E.Z. and Cone R.A. (1974) Rhodopsin: Light activated release of calcium. Fed. Proc. 33, 1471.

Tomita T. (1972) Light induced potential and resistance changes in vertebrate photoreceptor, in: Handbook of Sensory Physiology, Vol. VII/2 Physiology of Photoreceptor Organs (Fuortes M.G.M. ed.) pp. 483-511, Springer Verlag, Berlin.

Weller M., Vermaux N. and Mandel P. (1975) Role of light and rhododopsin phosphorylation in control of permeability of retinal rod outer segment disks to calcium ion. Nature 256, 68-70.

Yoshikami S. and Hagins W.A. (1973) Control of the dark current in vertebrate rods and cones, in: Biochemistry and Physiology of Visual Pigments (Langer H. ed.) pp. 245-255, Springer Verlag, Berlin.

CHAPTER 4

TAURINE, A PUTATIVE TRANSMITTER IN RETINA

P. Mandel, H. Pasantes-Morales and P.F. Urban

Centre de Neurochimie du CNRS, 11 Rue Humann
67085 Strasbourg Cedex, France

Present address Dr. H. Pasantes-Morales: Departamento de Biologia Experimental, Instituto de Biologia, Universidad Nacional Autonoma de Mexico, Mexico City
Dr. P.F. Urban is Chargé de Recherche au CNRS.

INTRODUCTION

Although taurine has been known as a constituent of different organs and tissues in invertebrate and vertebrate species, little was known until recently about its physiological role. The high levels of taurine present in retina as well as its strong depressant effect on retinal cell activity (Pasantes-Morales et al., 1972b; Bonaventure et al., 1974) make it a good candidate for a neurotransmitter role in this organ.

The accepted criteria for the identification of central nervous system transmitters state that a neurotransmitter candidate should:

a) be present and synthetized within the neurons and especially presynaptic nerve endings from which it is suspected of being released upon the arrival of a nerve impulse.
b) reproduce a specific event of synaptic transmission, excitatory or inhibitory, as well as the ionic membrane process evoked by the transmitter action, when added exogenously.
c) interact in the same way as the natural transmitter with an agent which blocks postsynaptic receptors.
d) be released to the extracellular fluid in response to stimulation of nerve terminals.
e) be rapidly inactivated after its physiological action at the synaptic level.

In the present chapter we shall discuss data in the light of the above criteria which support the hypothesis that one function of taurine in retina is to act as an inhibitory neurotransmitter.

OCCURRENCE AND DISTRIBUTION

Taurine is present in high levels in the retina of all species studied (Pasantes-Morales et al., 1972a; Starr, 1973) in spite of the striking differences existing in the structural and physiological organization of this organ between species (Dowling, 1970). The concentration of taurine in retina varies between 10-14 μmoles per g (Pasantes-Morales et al., 1972a; Starr, 1973) and accounts for about 50% of the total amount of free amino acids. In contrast to what is observed in brain (Levi and Morisi, 1971), taurine levels in retina do not decrease with development. In the chick retina, a transient decrease in taurine levels prior to the appearance of the electroretinogram (ERG) is immediately followed by a rapid rise, to attain the adult levels in the first days of post-hatching age (Pasantes-Morales et al., 1973b). In rat retina, an increase in taurine levels is observed during postnatal development (Macaione et al., 1974).

The localization of endogenous taurine in the different cell layers of the retina has not been extensively studied. The diffusibility of taurine makes this type of investigation a very difficult task. The separation of different regions of retina by microdissection is probably the most suitable method for the study of the distribution of soluble compounds within retinal cells. By using this technique, Kennedy and Voaden (1974) analysed the taurine content of the photoreceptor layer of the frog retina in comparison with the remaining retinal structures. They found that a high proportion of taurine in the whole retina is concentrated in this layer. However, technical limitations make it very difficult to determine the taurine concentration within the different layers of the retina, especially the layer of the nerve terminals.

The localization of exogenous taurine, taken up by the retina _in vitro_, could give some indication on the endogenous distribution of taurine, if the assumption is made that exogenous taurine is homogeneously mixed with the endogenous stores. However, the results on the distribution of ^{35}S-taurine in rabbit retina reported by Ehinger (1973) are at variance with those of Kennedy and Voaden (1974). In rabbit retina exogenous taurine seems to be mainly localized in the glial cells (Ehinger, 1973). This discrepancy may be explained by assuming the existence of a taurine uptake mechanism localized in the glial cells. The sites of endogenous stores and the compartment of physiologically active taurine would then not necessarily coincide with the localization of this uptake mechanism. Alternatively, species differences might explain the differences in the observed results; e.g., it is well known that GABA mainly accumulates in the amacrine cells of the frog and chick retina (Marshall and Voaden, 1974), whereas in rat retina it is mainly taken up by the glial cells (Neal and Iversen, 1972).

BIOSYNTHESIS

In animal tissues taurine may be formed along five different pathways (Gaitonde, 1970). The preferential pathway in nervous tissue seems to be the oxidation of cysteine to cysteine sulfinic acid, which by subsequent decarboxylation and further oxidation forms hypotaurine and taurine respectively (Peck and Awapara, 1967 ; Rassin and Gaull, 1975). This biosynthetic pathway is most probably also present in retina. A cysteine oxidase activity has been described in rat retina, exhibiting the same properties as the enzyme in brain (Di Giorgio et al., 1975). Cysteine sulfinate decarboxylase activity has also been detected in rat and chick retina. The study of the properties of cysteine sulfinate decarboxylase activity in chick retina also indicates a great similarity between the retinal and the brain enzyme. Cysteine sulfinate decarboxylase in chick retina is highly stimulated by pyridoxal phosphate, as has been reported for the enzyme in brain. In contrast, the liver enzyme is saturated with the cofactor.

The study of cysteine sulfinate decarboxylase activity during postnatal development of rat retina and during embryogenesis in chicks has shown that the enzyme activity increases noticeably in a relatively short period. Cysteine sulfinate decarboxylase activity in chicken retina increases from 0.78 to 1.91 μmole of substrate decarboxylated/h/g of wet weight, between the 10th and the 20th day of embryonic development. From hatching to adult age the increase observed is only from 2.28 to 2.55 μmoles/h/g (Fig. 4.1). A similar phenomenon occurs in rat retina, where the increase in cysteine sulfinate decarboxylase activity is from 1.85 at 10 days of postnatal development to 5.88 μmoles per g at 30 days of age (Fig. 4.1). Interestingly, the most noticeable change in the enzyme activity occurs in the critical periods of the development of the retina in each species and essentially parallels the morphological and functional maturation of the visual function. In the chick, the time of appearance of the ERG has been reported to be between the 16th and the 18th day of embryonic life (Witkovski, 1963). In the rat, the ERG appears after the 12th day and attains the adult size and form at about the 18th day of postnatal life (Dowling and Sidman, 1962). Therefore, changes in the activity of the enzyme may reflect the morphological differentiation of the

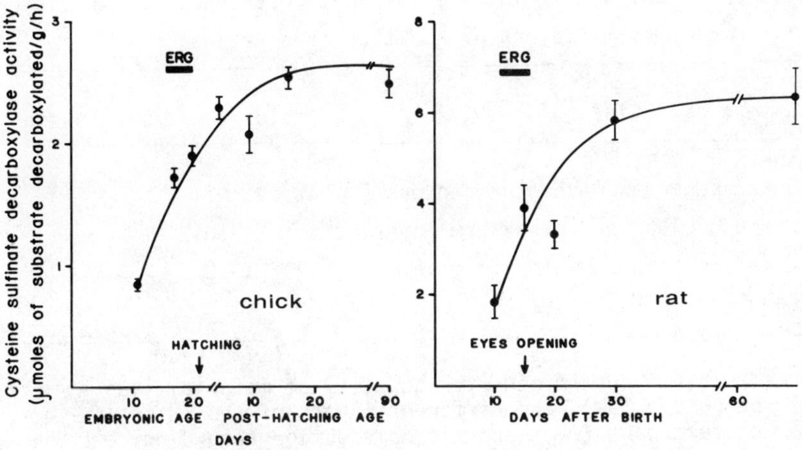

Fig. 4.1. Cysteine sulfinate decarboxylase activity in the retina of chick and rat during development. The enzyme activity was assayed by measuring the radioactivity of the $^{14}CO_2$ released from carboxyl-^{14}C cysteine sulfinic acid in retina homogenates (10% w/w), prepared in 0.067 M phosphate buffer (pH 6.8). The incubation mixture contained 33 mM neutralized cysteine sulfinic acid, 0.2-0.4 μCi of labeled cysteine acid, 10^{-4} M pyridoxal phosphate, 0.067 M phosphate buffer (pH 6.8) and 0.4 ml homogenate. Incubation time was 60 min. The results are means ± S.E.M. of 4-12 separate determinations.

synaptic contacts and the establishment of functional activity (Fig. 4.1).

In agreement with the above results, the distribution of cysteine sulfinate decarboxylase activity in adult chicken retina in different layers separated by microdissection shows that the enzyme is absent in the outer segments of photoreceptors (Table 4.1), whereas it appears concentrated in the cells making synaptic contacts (Mathur et al., 1975). Similar results are obtained after chemical subfractionation of retina: more than 50% of the cysteine sulfinate decarboxylase activity is recovered in the nerve ending fraction. When the inner synaptic layer of retina is degenerated by injection of monosodium glutamate in 10-day-old animals for a period of 10 days (Cohen et al., 1973), a substantial decrease (55%) of the cysteine sulfinate decarboxylase activity is observed. All these results are consistent with an association of the biosynthetic routes of taurine to synaptic terminals in the retina, which

Table 4.1. Distribution of cysteine sulfinate decarboxylase in different layers of adult chicken retina

Layers of retina	10^{-9}moles CO_2/h/mg protein
Outer segments of photoreceptors	Nil
Outer nuclear and plexiform layer	10.2
Inner nuclear and plexiform layer	18.5
Ganglion cells	N.D.

N.D.: not determined (the quantity of material available being too low). The different layers of the retina were dissected by free hand microdissection according to Lowry et al. (1956). The homogenates of the microdissected material were incubated for 30 min at 37°C in 5 mM of cold cysteine sulfinate and 1 μCi of ^{14}C-cysteine sulfinate labeled at the carboxyl group; the liberated $^{14}CO_2$ was counted in the Intertechnique liquid scintillation spectrometer model SL 30.

suggests a participation of this amino acid in the synaptic function.

PHYSIOLOGICAL ACTIONS

Taurine exerts a powerful depressant effect on the bioelectrical response of retinal cells. Intravitreal injections of taurine induce a rapid and strong inhibition on the b wave amplitude of the ERG (Pasantes-Morales et al., 1973a). The effect on taurine is specifically exerted on the distal electrical response of the retina; under no circumstances have modifications of the a wave been observed after taurine injection (Pasantes-Morales et al.,1973a). The maximum inhibitory effect of taurine is observed at concentrations within the range of physiological levels of taurine in retina (6 μmoles/g). This distinguishes the effects of taurine from those of other amino acids,like glycine or GABA,which also exert an inhibitory action on retinal activity. The amounts of GABA, required to abolish the b wave amplitude to the same extent as observed for taurine, are considerably higher than those present in the tissue and more than 3-fold higher than those of taurine (Pasantes-Morales et al., 1973a).

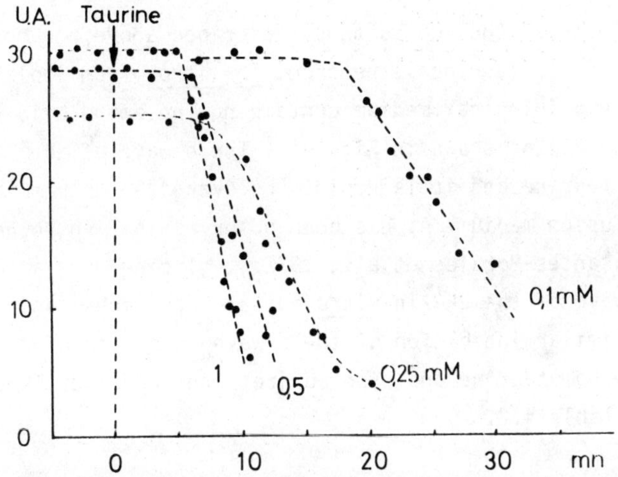

Fig. 4.2. Dose-effect relationship of the action of various taurine concentrations on electric responses to light stimulation of an isolated superfused retina. Perfusion is done at a flow rate of 3.5 ml medium per min. Ordinate: V, voltage amplitude in relative units. Abscissa: time of perfusion in minutes. Composition of the superfusion fluid: 80 mM NaCl, 2 mM KCl, 0.1 $MgCl_2$, 0.1 mM $CaCl_2$, 15 mM phosphate buffer (pH 7.8) and 5 mM glucose.

Table 4.2. EFFECT OF VARIOUS COMPOUNDS ON THE ERG OF FROG RETINA DURING PERFUSION

Compound	Formula	Concentration* mM
Taurine = 2 amino-ethane-sulfonic acid	$H_2N-CH_2-CH_2-SO_3H$	0.1
Gaba = 4-amino-butyric acid	$H_2N-CH_2-CH_2-CH_2-COOH$	0.15
Glycine	H_2N-CH_2-COOH	0.25
Cysteine sulfinic acid	$H_2N-CH(COOH)-CH_2-SO_2H$	0.5
l-Glutamic acid	$H_2N-CH(COOH)-CH_2-CH_2-COOH$	0.5
Hypotaurine = 2 amino-ethane sulfinic acid	$H_2N-CH_2-CH_2-SO_2H$	1
β-alanine	$H_2N-CH_2-CH_2-COOH$	1
Homotaurine = 3-amino-propane-sulfonic acid	$H_2N-CH_2-CH_2-CH_2-SO_3H$	1
Aspartic acid	$H_2N-CH(COOH)-CH_2-COOH$	5
Phenylalanine	$H_2N-CH(CH_2-C_6H_5)-COOH$	20

* Lowest concentration of amino acids producing a reduction in the b wave amplitude of the ERG of an isolated perfused frog retina

Identical effects on the ERG to those described above are observed when the retinal response to taurine is recorded _in vitro_, from isolated retina perfused with a physiological medium containing the amino acid (Pasantes-Morales et al., 1972c),as shown in Fig. 4.2. The b wave of the ERG is completely abolished by taurine and it is rapidly recovered after removal of taurine from the perfusion medium. As has been observed _in vivo_, other amino acids like GABA (Pasantes-Morales et al., 1972c), glycine or β-alanine also inhibit the b wave of the ERG _in vitro_ but at much higher dosages (Urban et al., 1975). Similar inhibition of the b wave is obtained when analogs of taurine, like homotaurine and hypotaurine, are perfused. These findings are presented in Table 4.2.

Studies on the localization of exogenous taurine at the subcellular structures of retina are consistent with a role for taurine in synaptic transmission in retina: at the moment of maximum effect on the b wave, the intravitreally injected taurine has been found concentrated in the inner synaptic layer, and most of it disappears from these sites when a normal ERG is recovered. In further support of this involvement of taurine in the inhibitory mechanisms of retina, the tectal evoked responses (Fig. 4.3) and the unit activities of the ganglion cells (Bonaventure et al., 1975) recorded after intravitreal injections of taurine show a progressive decrease leading to a total disappearance concurrent with the inhibition of the b wave amplitude

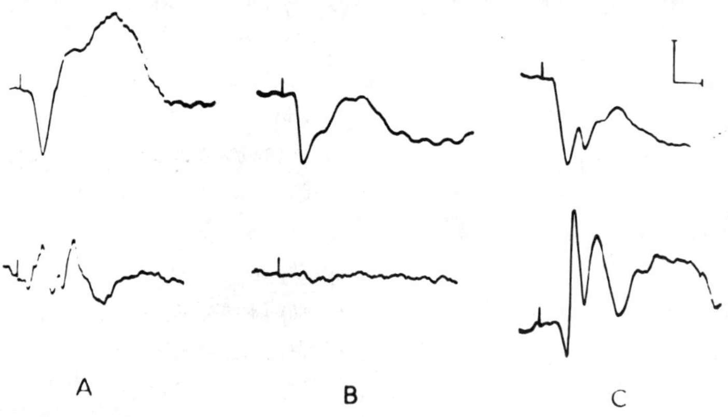

Fig. 4.3. Electroretinogram (upper traces) and tectal evoked responses (lower traces) before and after intravitreal injection of 0.3 M taurine. A: before, B: 1 h. after, C: 3 h. after injection. The calibration lines indicate 25 msec and 100 μV. Stimulation artifact (vertical lines) is given on each trace (Bonaventure et al, 1975).

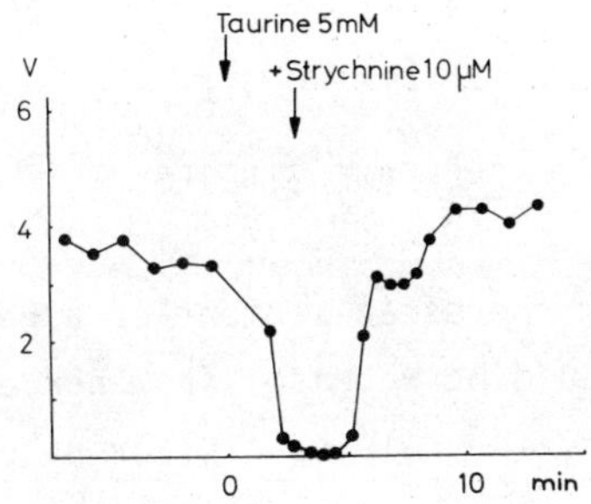

Fig. 4.4. Effect of taurine and of strychnine on the b wave amplitude of the electroretinogram of isolated perfused retina. Ordinate: V, voltage amplitude in relative units. Abscissa: perfusion time in minutes. Composition of the normal perfusion medium: see legend to Fig. 4.2. Successive additions during perfusion: at time zero 5 mM taurine, 3 min later 10 μM strychnine.

(Bonaventure et al.,1974). Thus taurine seems to be effectively blocking the transmission of visual information. The inhibition of the tectal evoked potential is also observed after injection of GABA, but whereas the effect of GABA on tectal evoked potentials closely parallels that on the ERG, the depressant effect of taurine on ERG persists after the recovery of the tectal potentials (Bonaventure et al., 1974), suggesting that the action of taurine in the retina may not be restricted to an effect on synaptic transmission.

The depressant effect of taurine on ERG is antagonized by strychnine. When strychnine is injected at the time of maximal depression of the b wave produced by taurine the effect is completely reversed. Furthermore, when strychnine is injected simultaneously to taurine, the depressant effect of taurine is markedly reduced or it is even absent (Bonaventure et al., 1974). Fig. 4.4 shows that the same results are obtained *in vitro* in the presence of strychnine in the perfusion medium (Urban and Dreyfus, 1974).

Picrotoxin or bicuculline, which are antagonists of the depressant effect of GABA on neuronal activity have no effect on the inhibitory action of taurine on ERG, suggesting that the effect of taurine is on another receptor than that of GABA (Bonaventure et al., 1974).

RELEASE STUDIES

An important criterion for the establishment of a neurotransmitter role for a substance is that it should be released from nerve terminals as a result of presynaptic stimulation. The release of taurine by procedures which are known to cause depolarization of nerve cells has been described for the retina. Stimulation of the retina by electrical impulses highly enhances the release of taurine; an increase of ^{35}S-taurine in the perfusion medium of about 10-fold the prestimulation value is observed after application of the electrical stimulus. Under identical conditions, the release of GABA is increased by about 3-fold, whereas the efflux of leucine is only slightly modified (Pasantes-Morales et al., 1974a). Another procedure for studying the stimulation of transmitter release by nerve cell depolarization is by increasing the potassium concentration in the extracellular medium. This is probably a more reliable method than the electrically induced depolarization, since it avoids the problems of variations in the current path and damage of the tissue by excessive electrical stimulation. The efflux of putative neurotransmitter substances has been reported to be significantly enhanced in the presence of a high potassium concentration. In the retina this condition is known to increase the release of GABA (Voaden and Starr, 1972). It also increases the efflux of taurine (Fig. 4.5). Raising the potassium concentration to 30 mM induces an increase in taurine release of about 50% over the resting efflux; 60 mM potassium produces an increase of 142% and 100 mM potassium enhances taurine release by more than 180%.

The most interesting result concerning the release of taurine is probably the demonstration of its increased efflux after illumination of the retina. When retinae loaded with ^{35}S-taurine and perfused at a high flow rate with a physiological medium are stimulated by flashes, the spontaneous efflux of labeled taurine is markedly increased (Pasantes-Morales et al., 1973c). This effect of light is observed in chick retina as well as in rat retina, in spite of their differençes in complexity and functional organization. Moreover, when newborn chickens are maintained in darkness, an accumulation of taurine in the retina is observed. In addition, after injection of radioactive ^{35}S-taurine the decrease of the amount of radioactive taurine present

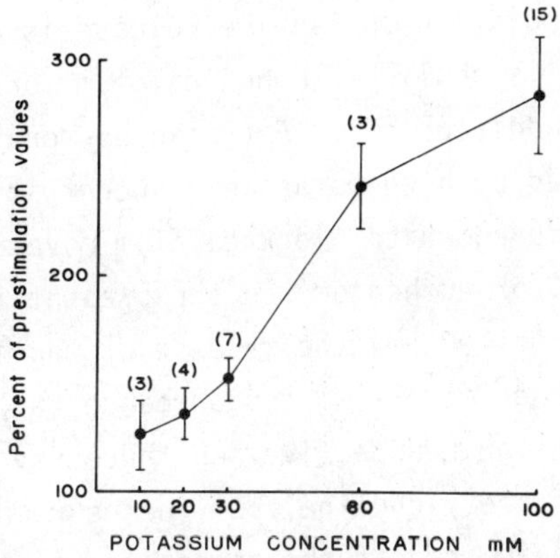

Fig. 4.5. Effect of potassium concentration on the efflux of ^{35}S-taurine from chick retina. Retinae of dark-adapted animals were loaded with ^{35}S-taurine in Krebs-bicarbonate buffer (2.5 μCi/ml), washed and transferred to incubation flasks containing 2 ml of medium containing 47 mM KCl, 28 mM NaCl and 100 mM choline chloride. The flasks were incubated at 37°C under continuous shaking; retinae were transferred every 5 min to series of vials containing 2 ml of warmed, oxygenated medium. After 20 min of incubation, stable efflux conditions were obtained and retinae were transferred to media containing the indicated concentrations of KCl, maintaining a constant osmolarity by reducing the choline chloride concentration. The taurine efflux was calculated as efflux rate constant and the maximum efflux rate constant achieved during 5 min exposure to various concentrations of potassium was expressed as the percentage of the efflux rate constant obtained just before stimulation. Results are means ± S.E.M. (vertical bars) of the number of experiments indicated in parentheses.

in the retina was much slower in dark-maintained animals (Pasantes-Morales et al., 1973b).

Illumination of the retina seems to affect specifically the efflux of taurine; studies on the effect of light on the release of other amino acids like GABA, glycine and glutamic acid have shown no effect at all, or only a slight stimulation.

Most neurohumoral release mechanisms are calcium-dependent. The stimulation of taurine release from the retina evoked by illumination, electrical pulses or high potassium concentration seems to be a calcium-dependent process. The effect of electrical stimulation on taurine release is considerably reduced, and that of illumination is abolished, when calcium ions are removed from the perfusion medium by the addition of EDTA (Pasantes-Morales et al., 1974a). Taurine release stimulated by high potassium concentration is very sensitive to the action of compounds known to block calcium movements across biological membranes. When verapamil or ruthenium red are present in the incubation medium at concentrations of 100 μM, the release of taurine evoked by high potassium is abolished. The latter two drugs reduce the calcium-dependent release of neurotransmitters or neuroactive substances by blocking calcium movements. The release of acetylcholine from the neuromuscular junction is markedly reduced by ruthenium red at the same concentration used in the experiments with the retina (Rahaminoff and Alnaes, 1973). Similarly, verapamil considerably decreases the release of biogenic amines from the cerebral cortex (Yarbrough et al., 1974) and that of neurohormones from the neurohypophysis (Eto et al., 1974).

The involvement of calcium ions in the mechanism of transmitter release has recently been confirmed by the use of compounds able to translocate calcium across a variety of biological membranes. The calcium ionophores, X537A and A23187, induce a marked increase in the release of acetylcholine from the neuromuscular junction (Kita and Van der Kloot, 1974), of norepinephrine from adrenergic neurons (Thoa et al., 1974) and of dopamine from synaptosomes (Holz, 1975). These substances also transport calcium into the retinal cells and most probably mediate the release of certain amino acids from the retina by this effect. X537A and A23187 stimulate the release of GABA, glycine and taurine without affecting that of leucine (Pasantes-Morales et al., 1974b; Salceda and Pasantes-Morales, 1975). The calcium ionophores evoke a release of taurine from the retina, which is considerably higher than that of GABA or glycine. Whereas the increase of the taurine efflux is stimulated by 70-90% in the presence of X537A or A32187, the release of GABA and glycine is stimulated by only 20-25%.

INACTIVATION OF TAURINE

A catabolic pathway, rapid enough to be responsible for the inactivation of taurine after its eventual action at the synaptic level, does not seem to exist. Such inactivation most probably takes place, as for most neurotransmitters, by means of a high affinity uptake mechanism. This kind of taurine transport system has been described in brain cortical slices (Pasantes-Morales et al., 1972b; Starr and Voaden, 1972) and more specifically in nerve endings isolated from this region (Dolara et al., 1972). In the retina of chick (Dolara et al., 1973), rat (Huxtable and Bressler, 1973) and rabbit (Ehinger, 1973) a transport system for taurine has been reported, which shows the properties currently ascribed to neurotransmitter transport systems. The uptake of taurine in the retina is highly dependent on sodium ions, temperature and metabolic energy, and is highly specific. The localization of the cellular sites, where this uptake of taurine occurs, has not yet been studied extensively. A report of Ehinger using autoradiographic techniques indicates, however, that taurine accumulated by this high affinity transport mechanism is concentrated at the Muller cells, the glial elements of the retina (Ehinger, 1973).

CONCLUDING REMARKS

The observations described here, when taken together, are highly suggestive of a transmitter role for taurine in retina. Most of the criteria required for neurotransmitters are fulfilled by taurine. Probably more vigorous tests of identity of action should be provided, involving comparisons of the potentials and conductance changes exerted on the postsynaptic membrane during synaptic activation and during application of taurine at specific synapses.

The demonstration of taurine release processes in isolated nerve endings could also provide more direct evidence for its participation in the synaptic functioning. Finally, the determination by sensitive histoautoradiographic methods of the intraneuronal taurine distribution might confirm its presence in the axon terminals, from where it could be released upon arrival of nerve impulse.

It should also be kept in mind that the amount of taurine in brain is rather high (Mark and Mandel, 1964), and that several reports concerning the distribution (Guidotti et al., 1972; Cutler and Dudzinki, 1974), the release, the uptake (Kandora et al., 1968) and the metabolism of taurine in brain are in agreement with a transmitter role. Thus taurine is unevenly distributed in the central nervous system (Agrawal et al., 1971; Perry et al., 1971) like GABA and glycine, which have been postulated as neurotransmitters. High concentrations of taurine were found in synaptic vesicles isolated from rat cerebral cortex (DeBelleroche and Bradford, 1973), although it was not confirmed for guinea pig cerebral cortex (Rassin, 1972).

The heterogeneity in the regional and cellular distribution of taurine as well as the differences observed in taurine decrease in the different regions during development, may be correlated with a functional role of this amino acid in nervous tissues.

Taurine is also a very effective depressor of the firing of neurons in brainstem and medulla oblongata (Curtis et al., 1968). The inhibitory effects of taurine on spinal neurons are antagonized by strychnine, and by strychnine as well as bicuculline in cortical neurons (Haas and Hosli, 1973). The release of endogenous taurine from cat cerebral cortex increases during stimulation of midbrain reticular formation (Jasper and Koyama, 1969). Kaczmarek and Adey (1974) confirmed this observation, showing an enhanced release of taurine in response to an increase of activity. Moreover, taurine is released from brain cortical and spinal cord slices in response to a depolarizing stimulus or electric stimulation (Kaczmarek and Davison, 1972; Kaczmarek and Adey, 1974). Finally, an active system of biosynthesis and inactivation of released taurine exists in the central nervous system (Jacobsen and Smith, 1968).

A role of taurine in retinal functions other than synaptic transmission may also be considered. An effect of taurine on calcium transport in biological systems has been suggested on the basis of experiments of Dolara et al. (1972, 1973). An action of taurine on potassium transport has also been suggested. These effects have not been studied in nervous tissue, but the possibility exists that the inhibitory effects of taurine on neuronal activity may be accounted for by changes in membrane permeability or in ionic gradients caused by the amino acid. A possible action of taurine on calcium movements in retina is of considerable interest in view of the critical role, which seems to be played by calcium transport in the phenomena which lead to the hyperpolarization of photoreceptors by light (see ch. 3 of this book). Studies of the effect of taurine on the kinetics of calcium transport at photoreceptor levels could give some indication on a possible involvement of taurine in this aspect of retinal physiology.

REFERENCES

Agrawal H.C., Davison A.N. and Kaczmarek L.K. (1971) Subcellular distribution of taurine and cysteine sulphinate decarboxylase in developing rat brain. Biochem. J. 122, 759-763

Bonaventure N., Wioland N. and Mandel P. (1974) Antagonists of the putative inhibitory transmitters of taurine and GABA in the retina. Brain Res. 80, 281-289

Bonaventure N., Bezaut M. and Wioland N. (1975) Taurine and GABA as putative neurotransmitters in the retina. First Europ. Neurosciences Meeting, Munich, Abstr. Exptl. Brain Res. suppl. 23, 47

Cohen A.I., McDaniel M. and Orr H. (1973) Absolute levels of some free amino acids in normal and biologically fractionated retinas. Invest. Ophthal. 12, 686-693

Curtis D.R., Hösli L. and Johnston G.A.R. (1968) A pharmacological study of the depression of spinal neurones by glycine and related amino acids. Exptl. Brain Res. 6, 1-18

Cutler R.W.P. and Dudzinski D.S. (1974) Regional changes in amino acid content in developing rat brain. J. Neurochem. 23, 1005-1009

DeBelleroche J.S. and Bradfors H.F. (1973) Amino acids in synaptic vesicles from mammalian cerebral cortex: a reappraisal. J. Neurochem. 21, 441-451

Di Giorgio R.M., Tucci G. and Macaione S. (1975) Cysteine oxidase activity in rat retina during development. Life Sci. 16, 429-436

Dolara P., Agresti A. and Pasquini G. (1972) Effect of taurine on calcium kinetic of guinea pig heart. Europ. J. Pharmacol. 24, 352-358

Dolara P., Marino P. and Buffani F. (1973) Effect of 2-amino ethanesulphonic acid (taurine) and 2-hydroxy ethansulphonic acid (isethionic acid) on calcium transport by rat liver mitochondria. Biochem. Pharmacol. 22, 2085-2094

Dowling J.E. and Sidman R.L. (1962) Inherited retinal dystrophy in the rat. J. Cell Biol. 14, 73-86

Dowling J.E. (1970) Organization of vertebrate retinas. Invest. Ophthal. 9, 651-680

Ehinger B. (1973) Glial uptake of taurine in the rabbit retina. Brain Res. 60, 512-516

Eto S., Wood J.M., Hutchins M. and Fleischer N. (1974) Pituitary $^{45}Ca^{++}$ uptake and release of ACTH, GH and TSH: effect of verapamil. Am. J. Physiol. 226, 1315-1320

Gaitonde M.K. (1970) Sulfur amino acids, in: Handbook of Neurochemistry "Metabolic Reactions in the Nervous System" (Lajtha A., ed.) Vol. III, pp. 225-287, Plenum Press, New York

Guidotti A., Badiani G. and Pepeu G. (1972) Taurine distribution in cat brain. J. Neurochem. 19, 431-435

Holz R. (1975) The release of dopamine from synaptosomes from rat striatum by the ionophores X537A and A23187. Biochim. Biophys. Acta 375, 138-152

Haas H.L. and Hösli L. (1973) The depression of brainstem neurones by taurine and its interaction with strychnine and bicuculline. Brain Res. 52, 399-402

Huxtable R. and Bressler R. (1973) Effect of taurine on a muscle intracellular membrane. Biochim. Biophys. Acta 323, 573-583

Jacobsen J.G. and Smith L.H. Jr. (1968) Biochemistry and physiology of taurine and taurine derivatives. Physiol. Rev. 48, 424-511

Jasper H.H. and Koyama I. (1969) Rate of release of amino acids from the cerebral cortex in the cats as effected by brainstem and thalamic stimulation. Canad. J. Physiol. Pharmacol. 47, 889-905

Kaczmarek L.K. and Davison A.N. (1972) Uptake and release of taurine from rat brain slices. J. Neurochem. 19, 2355-2362

Kaczmarek L.K. and Aday W.R. (1974) Factors affecting the release of ^{14}C-taurine from cat brain: the electrical effects of taurine on normal and seizure prone cortex. Brain Res. 76, 83-94

Kandora J., Levi G. and Lajtha A. (1968) Control of cerebral metabolite levels. II. Amino acid uptake and levels in various areas of the rat brain. Arch. Biochem. Biophys. 126, 249-260

Kennedy A.J. and Voaden M.J. (1974) Free amino acids in the photoreceptor cells of the frog retina. J. Neurochem. 23, 1093-1095

Kita H. and Van der Kloot W. (1974) Calcium ionophore X537A increases spontaneous and phasic quantal release of acetylcholine at frog neuromuscular junction. Nature 250, 658-660

Levi G. and Morisi G. (1971) Free amino acids and related compounds in chick brain during development. Brain Res. 26, 131-140

Lowry O.H., Roberts N.R. and Lewis C.H. (1956) The quantitative histochemistry of the retina. J. Biol. Chem. 220, 879-892

Macaione S., Ruggeri P., De Luca F. and Tucci G. (1974) Free amino acids in developing rat retina. J. Neurochem. 22, 887-891

Mark J. and Mandel P. (1964) Limites de l'homéostasie des acides aminés libres du système nerveux central du rat. C.R. Soc. Biol. 158, 2478-2481

Mathur R.L., Klethi J., Ledig M. and Mandel P. (1975) Cysteine sulfinate carboxylase in the visual pathway of adult chicken. Life Sci. in press.

Marshall J. and Voaden M. (1974) An autoradiographic study of the cells accumulating ^{3}H γ-aminobutyric acid in the isolated retinas of pigeons and chickens. Invest. Ophthal. 13, 602-607

Neal M.J. and Iversen L.L. (1972) Autoradiographic localization of ^{3}H-GABA in rat retina. Nature New Biol. 235, 217-218

Pasantes-Morales H., Klethi J., Ledig M. and Mandel P. (1972a) Free amino acids of chicken and rat retina. Brain Res. 41, 494-497

Pasantes-Morales H., Klethi J., Urban P.F. and Mandel P. (1972b) The physiological role of taurine in retina: uptake and effect on electroretinogram. Physiol. Chem. Phys. 4, 339-348

Pasantes-Morales H., Urban P.F., Klethi J. and Mandel P. (1972c) Etude de l'effet de la taurine sur l'électrorétinogramme de la rétine en perfusion. C.R. Acad. Sci. Paris Série D 275, 699-702

Pasantes-Morales H., Bonaventure N., Wioland N. and Mandel P. (1973a) Effect of intravitreal injections of taurine and GABA on chicken electroretinogram. Int. J. Neurosci. 5, 235-241

Pasantes-Morales H., Klethi J., Ledig M. and Mandel P. (1973b) Influence of light and dark in the free amino acid pattern of the developing chick retina. Brain Res. 57, 59-65

Pasantes-Morales H., Urban P.F., Klethi J. and Mandel P. (1973c) Light stimulated release of ^{35}S-taurine from chicken retina. Brain Res. 51, 375-378

Pasantes-Morales H., Klethi J., Urban P.F. and Mandel P. (1974a) The effect of electrical stimulation, light and amino acids on the efflux of ^{35}S-taurine from the retina of domestic fowl. Exptl. Brain Res. 19, 131-142

Pasantes-Morales H., Salceda R. and Gomez-Puyon A. (1974b) Effect of X537A on the release of amino acids in retina. Biochem. Biophys. Res. Commun. 58, 847-853

Peck E.J. and Awapara J. (1967) Formation of taurine and isethionic acid in rat brain. Biochim. Biophys. Acta 141, 499-506

Perry T.L., Berry K., Hansen S., Diamond S. and Mok C. (1971) Regional distribution of amino acids in human brain obtained at autopsy. J. Neurochem. 18, 513-519

Rahaminoff R. and Alnaes E. (1973) Inhibitory action of ruthenium red on neuromuscular transmission. Proc. Natl. Acad. Sci. USA 70, 3613-3616

Rassin D.K. (1972) Amino acids as putative transmitters: failure to bind to synaptic vesicles of guinea pig cerebral cortex. J. Neurochem. 19, 130-148

Rassin D.K. and Gaull G.E. (1975) Subcellular distribution of enzymes of transmethylation and transsulphuration in rat brain. J. Neurochem. 24, 969-978

Salceda R. and Pasantes-Morales H. (1975) A calcium coupled release of taurine from retina. Brain Res., in press.

Starr M.S. and Voaden M.J. (1972) The uptake, metabolism and release of ^{14}C-taurine by rat retina in vitro. Vision Res. 12, 1261-1269

Starr M.W. (1973) Effect of dark adaptation of the GABA system in retina. Brain Res. 59, 331-338

Thoa B., Costa J.L., Moss J. and Kopin I.J. (1974) Mechanism of release of norepinephrine from peripheral adrenergic neurons by the calcium ionophores X537A and A23187. Life Sci. II 14, 1705-1719

Urban P.F. and Dreyfus H. (1974) Données nouvelles sur le rôle de neurotransmetteur de la taurine dans la rêtine. J. Physiol. (Paris) 69, 303-304A

Urban P.F., Edel-Harth S. and Dreyfus H. (1975) Effet de divers acides aminés sur l'ERG de la rêtine en perfusion. J. Physiol. (Paris) 71, 166A

Voaden M.J. and Starr M.S. (1972) The efflux of radioactive GABA from rat retina in vitro. Vision Res. 12, 559-566

Witkovski P. (1963) An ontogenic study of retinal function in the chick. Vision Res. 3, 341-355

Yarbrough G.G., Lake N. and Phillis J.W. (1974) Calcium antagonism and its effect on the inhibitory actions of biogenic amines on cerebral cortical neurones. Brain Res. 67, 77-88

CHAPTER 5

GAMMA-AMINOBUTYRIC ACID AND GLYCINE AS RETINAL NEUROTRANSMITTERS

Mary J. Voaden

Department of Visual Science
Institute of Ophthalmology
Judd Street
London, WC1H 9QS

INTRODUCTION

It is now well recognized that the microiontophoretic application of γ-aminobutyric acid (GABA) or glycine to central nervous system (CNS) neurones will induce, usually, a hyperpolarising response based, possibly, on increased conductance of the neuronal membrane to chloride ions (Krjnevič, 1974; Curtis and Johnston, 1974). Moreover, in certain instances, stimulation of inhibitory inputs to such neurones produces membrane conductance changes which are very similar to the effects of GABA or glycine. Both amino acids are therefore considered as potentially acting in inhibitory neurotransmission. At presynaptic sites GABA may induce chloride conductance changes that lead to a depolarisation of the terminal (Nishi et al., 1974). The end result is again reduction of the excitatory signal but, this time, through diminution of transmitter release.

Retinal neurones have proved no exception to the general rule, and it is a consistent observation that the application of GABA or glycine to e.g. ganglion cells, either microiontophoretically or in the bathing medium, suppresses both spontaneous and light-induced electrical activity (see Graham, 1974). These effects are reversible.

Selectivity of response has been noted for CNS neurones in that cells in the spinal cord are more sensitive to glycine and those in the cerebral cortex or cerebellum to GABA (Krnjevič, 1974). Differential sensitivity has not yet been detected in studies on retinal neurones. An apparent lack of sensitivity to both amino acids was noted by Ames and Pollen (1969). However in these investigations the compounds were applied in the bathing medium. In studies where they have been tested iontophoretically on ganglion cells a considerably greater sensitivity has been found.

In the above work responses were recorded extracellularly so that membrane changes could only be inferred. However, in studies on the effects of GABA and glycine on horizontal cells of the carp retina, using intracellular recording, hyperpolarisation has been found (Murakami et al., 1972). The functional significance of these observations is unclear since, although horizontal cells may undergo hyperpolarising potential shifts during light stimulation of the retina, this is thought to be caused by the reduction of excitatory transmitter release from photoreceptor cells (cf. Dowling and Ripps, 1973). Intracellular recordings from other retinal neurones following the application of GABA or glycine have not been reported. It is known that both bipolar and amacrine cells may hyperpolarise on light stimulation of the tissue but this may be accompanied by an increase in the membrane resistance of these cells (Dowling, 1970; Toyoda, 1973; Toyoda et al., 1973).

Apart from the direct inhibitory effects of GABA and glycine on retinal neurones, antagonists of their actions will increase neuronal firing. For example, in the rabbit retina Ames and Pollen (1969) have reported that the glycine blocker strychnine, and sometimes the GABA antagonist picrotoxin, at levels which do not increase spontaneous activity, will induce firing in ganglion cells held under a light evoked inhibition. Additional effects of the GABA antagonists, picrotoxin and bicuculline are given on pages and further examples are cited by Graham (1974). With due caution as regards the specificity of available antagonists, because strychnine e.g. can also antagonise the action of taurine (cf. Mandel, ch. 4 of this book), there are, therefore, both direct and indirect indications for activity of these amino acids on retinal neurones.

In the cerebral cortex the actions of GABA and glycine are different in terms of effects on membrane conductance and reversal potentials (Kelly and Krnjević, 1969). If this proves true also in retinal cells, then it will be possible to distinguish their actions and to compare them with those of the natural transmitters at specific postsynaptic sites. Differentiation on the basis of sensitivity to specific antagonists is also possible. Experiments such as these are crucial to establishing GABA and glycine as retinal neurotransmitters and until they are done both amino acids can only be considered as potentially acting within the tissue.

A further necessity is to show that both compounds are present in retina to exert their actions. In the following sections, therefore, the endogenous concentrations and localisations of GABA and glycine, together with available information on the mechanisms maintaining them within retinas, will be discussed. Glycine and GABA will be dealt with separately.

GLYCINE

The levels of glycine found in retinas from a variety of species range from 0.60 - 4.00 μmoles/gm wet weight (Table 5.1).

Table 5.1. The concentration of glycine and γ-aminobutyric acid in retina

Species	Concentration (μmoles/gm wet wt.)				References
	GLYCINE		GABA		
	light	dark	light	dark	
Rat	2.30	2.52	1.92	1.93	Starr (1973)
	1.03		1.55		Pasantes-Morales et al. (1972)
	2.52		4.44		*Macaione et al. (1974)
	2.21		3.20		†Voaden et al., unpubl. observns.
Mouse	2.03	2.09	2.00	1.63	*Cohen et al. (1973)
Rabbit			0.51		*Kuriyama et al. (1968)
			1.21		Davis et al. (1969)
	3.21		3.54		†Voaden et al., unpubl. observns.
Chicken	2.01	2.00	3.69	3.43	Starr (1973)
	1.49		3.02		Pasantes-Morales et al. (1972)
Pigeon	4.00		3.81		†Voaden et al., unpubl. observns.
Frog	1.62	1.68	2.70	2.25	Starr (1973)
			3.48	1.39	*Graham et al. (1970)
	1.17		1.12		Kennedy and Voaden (1974a)
Goldfish	0.63	0.70	1.96	1.42	Starr (1973)
			3.15	1.65	Lam (1972)
Brain	0.55 - 1.45		0.83 - 2.27		McIlwain and Bachelard (1971)

*Recalculations based on 1 gm wet wt. = 0.12 gm protein
= 0.20 gm dry wt.

†For technique see Kennedy and Voaden (1974a).

No significant differences have been found between light or dark adapted tissue. In studies where the retina has been sectioned in a radial plane at

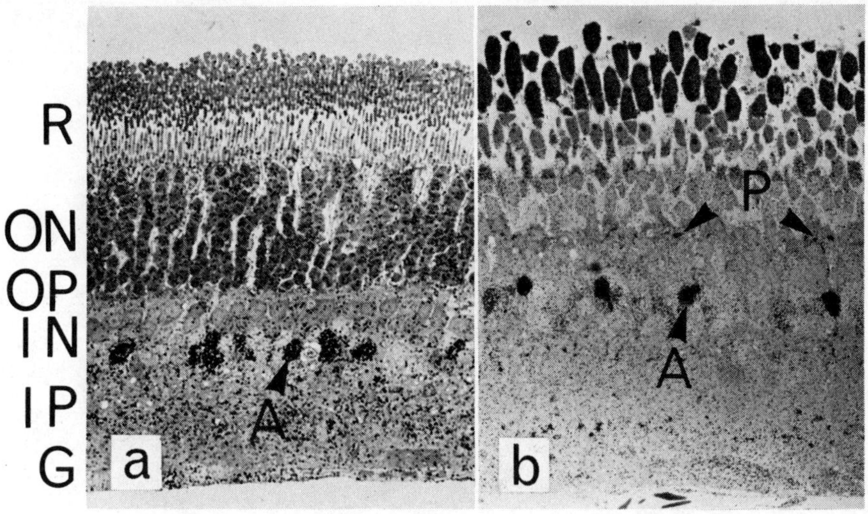

Fig. 5.1. Light microscope autoradiographs showing the uptake of ^{3}H-glycine into (a) rat retina (x350) and (b) frog retina (x410).
Retinas were incubated for 30 min. in Krebs bicarbonate medium (adjusted to 280 mOsm for frog), containing 1.46×10^{-5}M ^{3}H-glycine (100 μCi/ml). Incubation temperatures were 37°C for rat and 25°C for frog.
R-photoreceptor inner and outer limbs, ON-outer nuclear layer (photoreceptor nuclei), OP-outer plexiform (synaptic) layer, IN-inner nuclear layer, IP-inner plexiform layer, G-ganglion cell and nerve fibre layer.
In both species, glycine uptake has occurred into cells in the position of amacrine interneurones (A) and into the inner plexiform layer. In frog, grains are also present over the synaptic terminals of the photoreceptor cells (P). (Voaden et al., 1974, Marshall and Voaden, 1974a, 1975a).

the level of the outer plexiform (synaptic) layer (see Kennedy and Voaden, 1974a), 60-70% of the total endogenous glycine has been found in cells on the vitreal side of the photoreceptors. Frog, rat, rabbit and pigeon have been investigated (Kennedy and Voaden, 1974a; Voaden, Nathwani and Lake, unpublished observations). As yet a finer localization has not been reported. However, an alternative way to investigate the possible distribution of endogenous pools is to locate the sites able to accumulate the exogenously applied compound into the tissue, either by exchange or net uptake. When this is done for radioactive glycine, using autoradiography, it has been shown consistently in a variety of species that the label enters a population of cells on the inner side of the inner nuclear layer, a position characteristic of amacrine interneurones. Ganglion cells are also labeled to a varying extent. This has been studied in mammalian, avian and amphibian retinas (rat, cat, rabbit, guinea pig, monkey, human, pigeon, chicken and frog: Ehinger and Falck, 1971; Bruun and Ehinger, 1974; Marshall and Voaden, 1974a, b; Voaden et al., 1974). Examples of the pattern of uptake are shown in Fig. 5.1a and b.

In the frog retina (Fig. 5.1b) incorporation occurs also into the outer plexiform (synaptic) layer. E.M. autoradiography has shown that the uptake is localized over photoreceptor pedicles (Marshall and Voaden, 1975a). The significance of this finding is not known and it has not been observed in the other species so far investigated. However, it may prove pertinent that more endogenous glycine is found in the photoreceptor cell layer of the frog retina when the synaptic pedicles are included in the fraction than when they are omitted (cf. Kennedy and Voaden, 1974a, b).

Apart from the labeling of cell bodies of the inner nuclear layer, perhaps associated with amacrine cells, in most if not all species grains are present also over the inner plexiform layer, a region rich in nerve endings. As amacrine cells are the retinal interneurones that synapse in this layer of the retina and are thought to be involved in inhibitory modulation of the visual impulse, the uptake of radioactive glycine into both locales is of considerable interest. Significance is further increased by the fact that the uptake systems have properties suggested to be associated with neurotransmitter inactivation mechanisms (Krnjević, 1974; Curtis and Johnston, 1974). Thus, they are sodium dependent and temperature sensitive. Kinetic studies on retinas from rabbits (Bruun and Ehinger, 1972), rats (Neal et al., 1973), and frogs (Voaden et al., 1974) have shown that evidence can be obtained for two components to the transport systems, one with a "high" affinity for the amino acid (K_m about 10-20μM) and one with a K_m of approximately 1.0mM (Neal et al., 1973). The latter is in the range usually found for amino acid transport systems, including non-neuroactive compounds. It has been suggested that high affinity kinetics may correlate with the role of amino acids in neurotransmission. The rapid reuptake, possible in spite of low external concentrations, would serve to remove the amino acid from the extracellular spaces and to terminate its action (Iversen and Neal, 1968). In support of this idea a high affinity uptake has been reported for glycine in spinal cord, where it is thought to be a transmitter, but not in cerebral cortex, where it is not strongly neuroactive (Johnston and Iversen, 1971; Krnjević, 1974). The presence of such a high affinity system in retina can therefore be regarded as consistent with a possible neurotransmitter role for the amino acid. Studies on the frog retina suggest that the high affinity uptake system mediates net uptake and not merely exchange (Voaden et al., 1974).

In studies of compounds as neurotransmitters it is pertinent to ask how they are retained by the tissue under various conditions of stimulation. With the retina, the main condition of interest is that of light stimulation as compared with dark adaptation. Where total endogenous glycine levels have been measured, no differences have been found (Table 5.1). However, when dark adapted retinas have been preloaded with radioactive glycine and then light stimulated, an increased output of the radionuclide over its spontaneous efflux rate has been observed (Ehinger and Lindberg, 1974). This effect, which has been seen with retinas from cat and rabbit, is eliminated if calcium is removed from the superfusion medium and EDTA is added (Ehinger and Lindberg-Bauer, unpublished observations). This is a relevant observation as calcium dependence is frequently associated with the neural release of transmitters. In the above experiments the light source was a xenon flash tube, 15 cm from the retina and operated at 2 Hz. In a comparable study on the frog retina, a consistent increase in the output of glycine was not observed (Voaden, 1974), but stimulus parameters were less powerful.

The studies performed so far on glycine homeostasis in retinas can only be considered preliminary. They do, however, show that glycine is present, perhaps in specific amacrine cells, and that its efflux can be altered by a physiological stimulus. These facts alone make it worthy of consideration as a retinal inhibitory neurotransmitter.

γ-AMINOBUTYRIC ACID

The concentrations of GABA reported in retina are similar to those found in brain and are shown in Table 5.1. In the mouse, frog and goldfish the levels fall from between 7 and 57% on going from light to dark. In contrast, in the rat and chicken they remain the same on dark-adaptation. In the chicken, however, lower retinal levels are seen if the birds are reared in continuous darkness rather than in a normal day/night environment (Pasantes-Morales et al., 1973). No comparable changes have yet been reported for the rat retina. Species differences in response to light have been detected also in studies on the rate of incorporation of radio-labeled glucose carbon into the GABA molecule *in vivo* (Table 5.2; Starr,1975). Whereas in the frog there is a 36% increase in the light-stimulated as compared with the dark-adapted eye, in the rat retina the rates remain the same. The increased incorporation of radioactive carbon into GABA in the light-stimulated frog retina could result from the increased activity of glutamic decarboxylase (GAD) that has also been reported (Graham et al.,1970; Starr,1973). The concurrent decrease in radioactive glutamate, seen in Table 5.2,might follow as it is the precursor of GABA.

Table 5.2. The *in vivo* metabolism of ^{14}C-glucose by retinas from rat and frog

Product	Rat		Frog	
	dark	light	dark	light
Aspartate	386	409	303	339
Glutamate	1441	1388	3271	2582 ($p<0.01$)
Glutamine	525	511	1208	1417 ($p<0.01$)
γ-Aminobutyric acid	513	540	960	1306 ($p<0.001$)

Animals were fasted and dark-adapted overnight. They were then fitted with one opaque and one transparent contact lens and subjected to a white light of 20 μjoules, flashed for 30 min. at 2 Hz, duration 25 μsec. Frogs were injected intraperitoneally with 20 μCi ^{14}C-glucose and rats received 50 μCi ^{14}C-glucose via the femoral vein.
Each result is the mean of 24 experiments and is expressed as dpm/retina. Contralateral comparisons of results were made using the paired t-test: all S.E. lay in the range ±5-9%. (Taken from Starr, 1975).

The reasons for these species differences in the response of the GABA system to light are not known, but metabolic studies also suggest that GABA is handled very differently in these two types of retinas (see below).

Apart from effects of light on endogenous levels of GABA, studies on the release of the amino acid have also been undertaken. Using conditions similar to those in the glycine experiments discussed previously, i.e. preloading the tissue with radioactive GABA and following loss of the label, both in the presence and absence of inhibitors of GABA metabolism, no consistent changes in release rates have been observed. Rat, frog and chicken have been studied (Voaden and Starr, 1972; Kennedy and Voaden, 1974c; Pasantes-Morales et al., 1974). Pasantes-Morales and co-workers did produce a slight increase in output of radionuclide, from retinas preloaded with ^{14}C-GABA, on repeated stimulation of the chicken retina with light, but release was minimal compared with the effects on ^{35}S-taurine. No changes in the efflux rate of endogenous GABA from retinas on light stimulation have been observed, either in direct estimations (Pasantes-Morales et al., 1974; Neal, 1975) or when the pools are prelabeled with radioactive glucose (rat and frog: Starr, 1975).

Endogenous localization of GABA

Because of its ordered structure it is possible to slice the retina in a tangential plane and to obtain fractions enriched in specific cell types. The sections do not consist exclusively of specific cells however and all fractions from the inner to the outer limiting membrane contain Muller fibre cytoplasm, as these cells run in a radial plane through the tissue.

When sectioning has been done, the retinal layers are analysed for the enzyme synthetising GABA from glutamic acid, GAD (Fig.5.2a & b). Peak activity is found, in both rat and frog, in the inner plexiform (synaptic) fraction (Graham,1972,1974; Graham & Pong,1975). GABA is more widely distributed (Fig. 5.2c & d), but again peak levels are seen in the same region. Apart from the strong association of GABA with an area of retina known to have a high density of synaptic terminals there is also, in both species, evidence for a background level running through the tissue that could indicate a glial pool. If the major amount of GABA seen in the photoreceptor cell fractions is associated with the Muller fibres (which must occupy less than 40% of the fraction), the level reached in the cell could be quite high, particularly in the rat. However, GABA may also have a metabolic role in photoreceptors themselves. Histochemical studies have shown that the GABA bypath may be present in the inner limits of these cells, GABA-αoxoglutarate transaminase having been demonstrated in the rat retina (Hyde and Robinson, 1974) and succinic semialdehyde dehydrogenase in the tiger salamander (Moore and Gruberg, 1974).

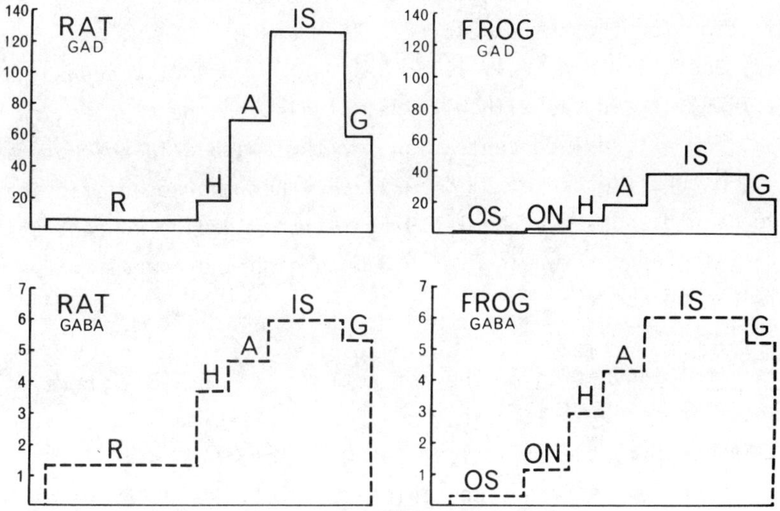

Fig. 5.2. The distribution of GABA and GAD through retinas of the rat and frog.
Dark adapted rats and frogs were decapitated and the heads frozen in petroleum ether and dry ice. Tangential sections (8μ) of the freed, frozen eyes were cut and lyophilized. The retina was then microdissected into five (rat) or six (frog) layers.
R-photoreceptor cells, OS-photoreceptor outer segments, ON-photoreceptor cell bodies, H-outer part of inner nuclear layer, rich in horizontal cells, A-inner part of inner nuclear layer, rich in amacrine cells IS-inner plexiform (synaptic) layer, G-ganglion cells and nerve fibres. The width of each layer has been approximated to its relative thickness within the whole retina.
GAD is expressed as μmoles GABA formed/hr/gm wet weight . retina and GABA as μmoles/gm wet weight retina.
(Data taken from Graham, 1974; see also Graham, 1972 and Graham and Pong, 1975).

Autoradiography

The similarities in the endogenous distribution of both GABA and GAD through rat and frog retinas contrast with the patterns of uptake of exogenously applied GABA as detected by autoradiography. In the rat retina *in vitro* (Fig. 5.3a) GABA is taken up predominantly by glial cells (Neal and Iversen, 1972; Marshall and Voaden, 1974a), whereas in the frog it enters into neurones (Fig. 5.3c; Voaden et al., 1974). Studies on the accumulation of GABA in these species have shown that, like glycine, it is taken up by energy- and sodium-dependent systems that are temperature sensitive and show both high and low affinity kinetics for the amino acid (K_{m1} 25μM and K_{m2} 250μM; Starr and Voaden, 1972; Goodchild and Neal, 1973; Neal et al., 1973; Voaden et al., 1974; Neal, 1975). Again, as with glycine, studies on the frog retina have implied that at low external concentrations of the amino acid net uptake rather than exchange occurs (Voaden et al., 1974). Further characteristics of these systems have been discussed by Neal (1975). At the loading concentrations used for the autoradiographs shown in Fig. 5.3 both high and low affinity "carriers" would be active.

Following *in vitro* incubation of the rat retina with ^{3}H-GABA, there is no clear evidence for neuronal labeling. However, 3 hrs after intraocular injection of the amino acid, there is clear uptake into cell bodies in the position of amacrine interneurones (Bruun and Ehinger, 1974). Glial uptake of ^{3}H-GABA also occurs *in vivo* and can be seen most readily in the early stages following the injection. It is not clear, therefore, whether amacrine labeling results from a transfer of radionuclide from glia to amacrine cells or whether both are labeled in the initial incorporation of ^{3}H-GABA. The ability to accumulate exogenously applied GABA appears to be a characteristic property of mammalian Muller fibres. It has been observed in a range of species including man and other primates (Bruun and Ehinger, 1974; Marshall and Voaden, 1975c). In some retinas, however, for example the cat (Fig. 5.3b) and rabbit, definite incorporation of ^{3}H-GABA into putative amacrine interneurones is also evident, even in short term *in vitro* experiments. Whether this is equivalent to the "amacrine" labeling seen in the rat remains to be investigated.

Comparing the pattern of GABA uptake seen in the rat retina (Fig. 5.3a) with that of the frog (Fig. 5.3c), the differences are immediately apparent, because in the latter species there is no evidence for uptake of GABA by the Muller fibres, but various types of neurones are labeled, including horizontal and amacrine cells. There is also some entry into ganglion cells and a heavy grain density over a subpopulation of bipolar cells. This observation is unexpected as bipolar cells are generally considered to be links in a direct excitatory pathway. However, their identity is confirmed by the observation that, occasionally, labeled Landolts clubs can be seen extending from them to the outer limiting membrane (Marshall and Voaden, unpublished observation). The autoradiograph in Fig. 5.3c is of a dark-adapted frog retina. The labeling of

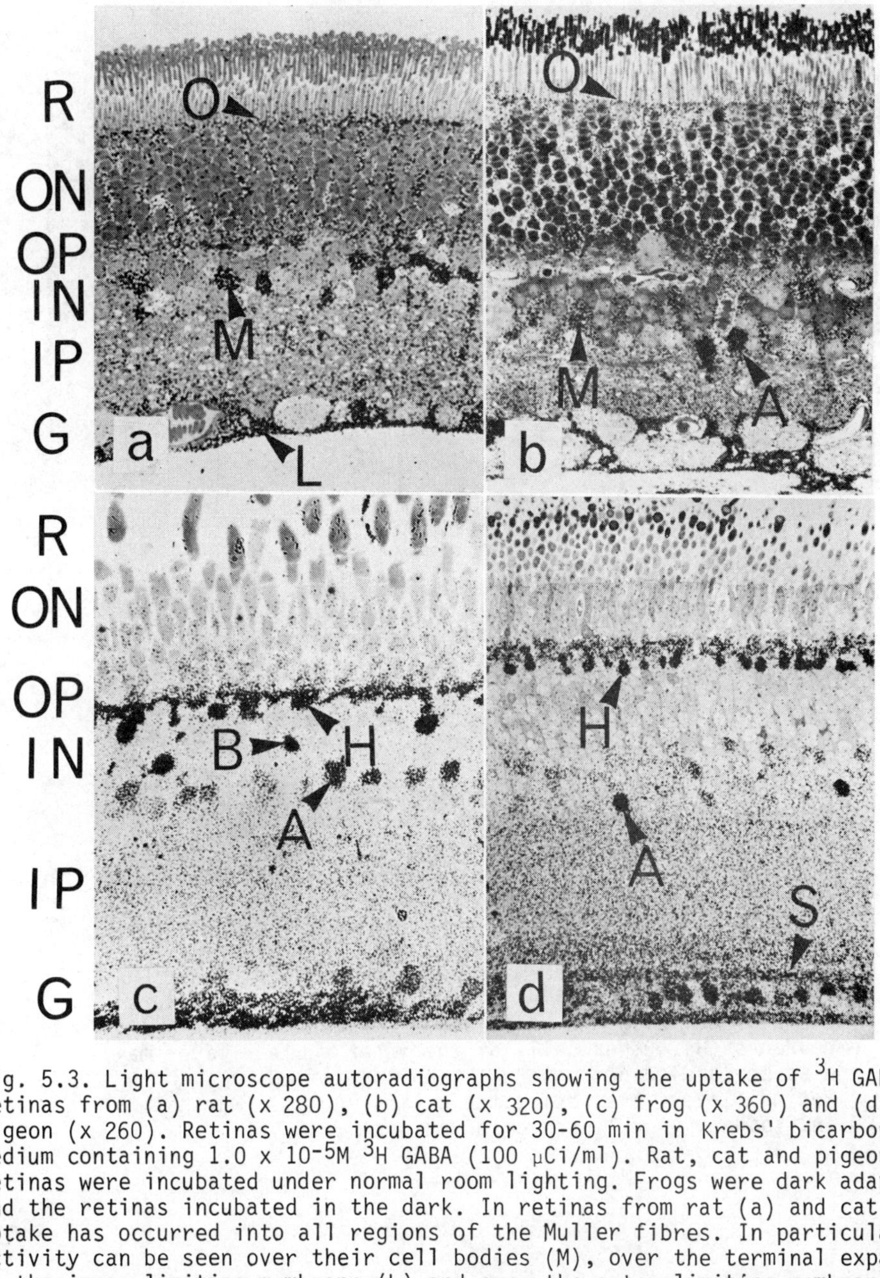

Fig. 5.3. Light microscope autoradiographs showing the uptake of ^{3}H GABA into retinas from (a) rat (x 280), (b) cat (x 320), (c) frog (x 360) and (d) pigeon (x 260). Retinas were incubated for 30-60 min in Krebs' bicarbonate medium containing 1.0 x 10^{-5}M ^{3}H GABA (100 μCi/ml). Rat, cat and pigeon retinas were incubated under normal room lighting. Frogs were dark adapted and the retinas incubated in the dark. In retinas from rat (a) and cat (b) uptake has occurred into all regions of the Muller fibres. In particular activity can be seen over their cell bodies (M), over the terminal expansions at the inner limiting membrane (L) and over the outer limiting membrane (O). In the cat retina, high grain density is present also over cells in the position of amacrine interneurones (A). In frog (c) and pigeon (d), ^{3}H GABA has entered into cells in the positions of horizontal (H) and amacrine (A) interneurones, and into the inner plexiform layer. In the frog retina bipolar cells (B) are also labeled. S-innermost synaptic region of the inner plexiform layer. Retinal layers are designated as in Fig. 5.1. (Marshall and Voaden, 1974a and c, 1975c; Voaden et al., 1974).

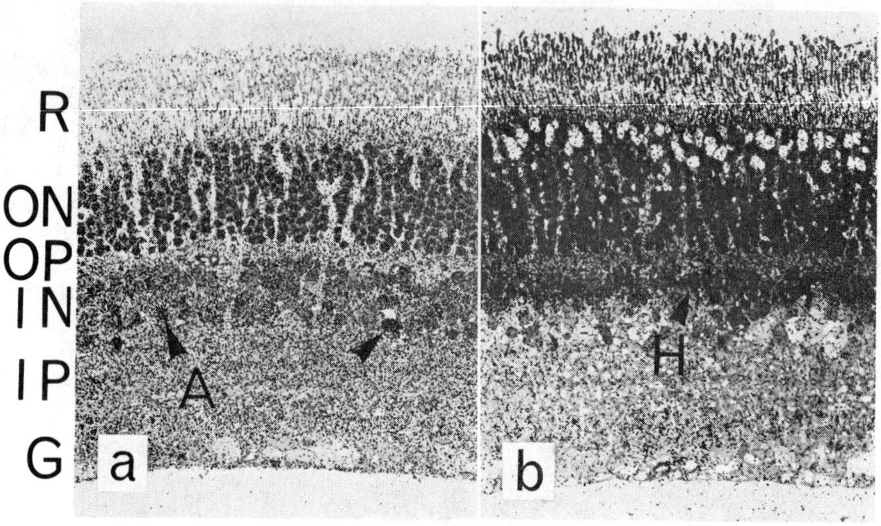

Fig. 5.4. Light microscope autoradiographs showing the uptake of (a) ^{3}H glutamine (x350) and (b) ^{14}C glucose (x350) by the rat retina in vitro. Retinas were incubated for 30 min at 37°C in Krebs bicarbonate buffer containing 5.5mM unlabeled glucose and equilibrated with 5% CO_2 in O_2: (a) one retina in 1.0 ml medium containing 100μCi ^{3}H glutamine (23Ci/m mol); (b) one retina in 0.1 ml medium containing 35μCi ^{14}C glucose (268mCi/m mol). Retinas were processed for autoradiography as described by Marshall and Voaden (1974a). They were fixed in glutaraldehyde followed by osmium textroxide and were embedded in Epon.

Following glutamine uptake, grains are distributed throughout the retina but heavier labeling is present over some cells in the position of amacrine interneurones (A). In retinas incubated with ^{14}C glucose, very heavy grain density is present over photoreceptors and over cells in the position of horizontal interneurones (H). Other cells of the inner nuclear layer may also be labeled but have not been identified.

Retinal layers are designated as in Fig. 5.1 (Marshall and Voaden, unpublished observations).

amacrine cells is less evident in the bleached tissue (Voaden et al., 1974), but it can be seen when 0.1 mM amino-oxyacetic acid is included in the medium (Marshall and Voaden, unpublished observation). This result is difficult to reconcile with the observation that GABA-transaminase activity in the frog retina is unaffected by the adaptational state of the tissue (Graham et al., 1970; Starr, 1973) and further studies are needed before it can be explained. A further effect of amino-oxyacetic acid on the frog retina is to eliminate the labeling of horizontal cell bodies by ^{3}H-GABA; radionuclides accumulating in this region in the untreated retina may therefore be metabolites of GABA.

The frog retina is not alone in showing a clear neuronal uptake of GABA. It has been reported also in goldfish (Lam and Steinman, 1971), chicken and pigeon retinas (Fig. 5.3d; Marshall and Voaden, 1974c). In these species there is no clear evidence for bipolar cell labeling, but there is incorporation of GABA into amacrine and horizontal cell bodies. In the pigeon and chicken, ganglion cells and strata of the inner plexiform layer are also clearly labeled (cf. Fig. 5.3d).

A further species difference is that horizontal cells in the dark-adapted goldfish retina are not heavily labeled by exogenously applied GABA (cf. Fig. 5.3c). They do, however, actively accumulate it when the tissue is light-stimulated (Lam and Steinman,1971). In the goldfish retina horizontal cell axons can synthetise GABA from L-glutamate (Lam,1975), and the concentration of endogenous GABA and its rate of synthesis are increased when the retina is light-stimulated (Lam,1972). Thus GABA is a serious candidate for an inhibitory neurotransmitter of horizontal cells in the goldfish - and, possibly, in frog, pigeon and chicken as well.

In mammalian retinas no association of GABA with horizontal cells has yet been established. However, we cannot rule out the possibility that it might be formed intracellularly from an endogenous substrate. In the rat retina, autoradiography has shown that although glutamine (cited as a GABA precursor *in vivo*, cf. Van den Berg, 1973) is not taken up specifically by horizontal cells (Fig. 5.4a), glucose *is* (Fig. 5.4b; Marshall and Voaden, unpublished observation). Moreover glucose is actively catabolised and GABA may be formed (cf. Table 5.2). Further studies are needed to see if this synthesis is occurring in horizontal cells. The autoradiographs shown in Fig. 5.4 are of retinas incubated for 30 min. with the radionuclides. Earlier (5 and 10 min. incubation) glutamine incorporation into the Muller fibres is more pronounced.

It would appear from the autoradiographic studies surveyed so far that in mammalian species GABA is taken up by glial cells, whereas in other vertebrates neuronal uptake predominates. However, similar studies on the elasmobranch skate retina have shown that in this species ^{3}H-GABA, as in the mammals, is taken up by the Muller fibres (H. Ripps, unpublished observation). Moreover the uptake is heavier in the light-stimulated retina than in the dark-adapted tissue. As yet we have no explanation for these species differences. However, it has been found that the majority of ganglion cells in the dogfish, a species closely related to skate, have antagonistic centre and surround responses (Stell et al., 1970, 1975). They, therefore, resemble more closely the response characteristics of the majority of ganglion cells in mammalian retinas, rather than the more complex response patterns seen, for example, in the frog and pigeon (Stell, 1972). It will be of interest to know the response characteristics of ganglion cells in the skate retina. Possible correlations between the functional organization of retinas and the pattern of GABA uptake have been discussed by Marshall and Voaden (1975c).

Metabolic organization

The close similarities in endogenous distribution and formation of GABA in rat and frog retinas, compared with the divergence in sites of uptake, suggest different organizations of GABA metabolism in these species.

Metabolic organization in the retina appears very similar to cerebral cortex in the following respect. When certain substrates, e.g. serine, leucine, glutamate, aspartate and bicarbonate, are metabolized by the tissue, glutamine is produced with a higher specific activity than the total tissue glutamate pool (Starr, 1974). As glutamate is the immediate precursor of glutamine, it must mean that the glutamine is being formed from a small glutamate pool of higher specific activity than the total, and that the substrate is feeding into this pool. Glucose does not show this labeling and appears to supply carbon atoms to most, if not all, glutamate pools. There is evidence for the presence of a "small" glutamate pool, active in the production of glutamine, in retinas from both rat and frog (Starr, 1974; Kennedy et al., 1974). In addition, autoradiography has shown that glutamate, which also feeds specifically into this pool, is in both species predominantly taken up by the Muller cells (Kennedy et al., 1974; Bruun and Ehinger, 1974). The implication is that glia are the major location of the "small" glutamate pool in retina, as is the case in the brain (Balázs et al., 1973).

GABA is a substrate generally recognized as feeding into the "small" glutamate compartment and, in brain, gives rise to glutamine of a higher specific activity than the total tissue glutamate (Balázs et al., 1973). However, when it is metabolized by retina, species differences are seen which may be correlated with the different sites of GABA uptake.

This has been studied (Voaden, Nathwani and Lake, unpublished observation) using a modification of the method described by Minchin and Beart (1975). Retinas are incubated for 60 min. in Krebs bicarbonate buffer (tonicity adjusted to 280 mOsm for the frog) containing 30 μCi/ml ^{14}C-GABA (232 mCi/mmol.). The incubation temperature is 37° C. for the mammalian and avian retinas and 25° C. for the frog. Individual portions (10-15 mg wet wt.) of retinal tissue are then weighed and homogenized in 1.0 ml 75% alcohol. Mixtures are centrifuged and the supernatants evaporated. Supernatant residues are reconstituted in 50 μl 0.05M sodium bicarbonate and portions dansylated with ^{3}H-dansyl chloride as described by Kennedy and Voaden (1974a). The dansylated amino acids are separated by thin-layer chromatography on micropolyamide plates and the individual spots (viewed under U.V. light) cut from the plate. Radioactivity is counted on a Packard 3375 liquid scintillation spectrometer, using the restricted ^{14}C and ^{3}H channels. Correction is made for background. crossover and efficiency of counting. Whereas all the tissue free amino acids are dansylated, and are, therefore, labeled with tritium, only those derived from ^{14}C-GABA contain radioactive carbon. The $^{14}C/^{3}H$ ratio of each sample is, therefore, a measure of the specific activity of the amino acid within the tissue.

The results (Fig. 5.5) show that in the rat and cat, where GABA enters predominantly into glial cells, the specific activity of glutamine exceeds that of glutamate (cf. Starr, 1974), but in frog and pigeon, where GABA uptake is neuronal (Fig. 5.3), the specific activity of the glutamine is considerably lower and is less than that of the total tissue glutamate. The present conclusions are at variance with those reached by Starr (1975).* However, in the latter study, the estimate for specific activity of the metabolites of GABA was based on endogenous levels present in the tissue in the absence of the labeled substrate. This might be an invalid approximation, as exogenous GABA could change endogenous amino acid levels.

The present results imply that in retinas from frog and pigeon GABA-carbon

*Starr, M.S., 1975, Biochem. Pharmacol. 24, 1193-1197.

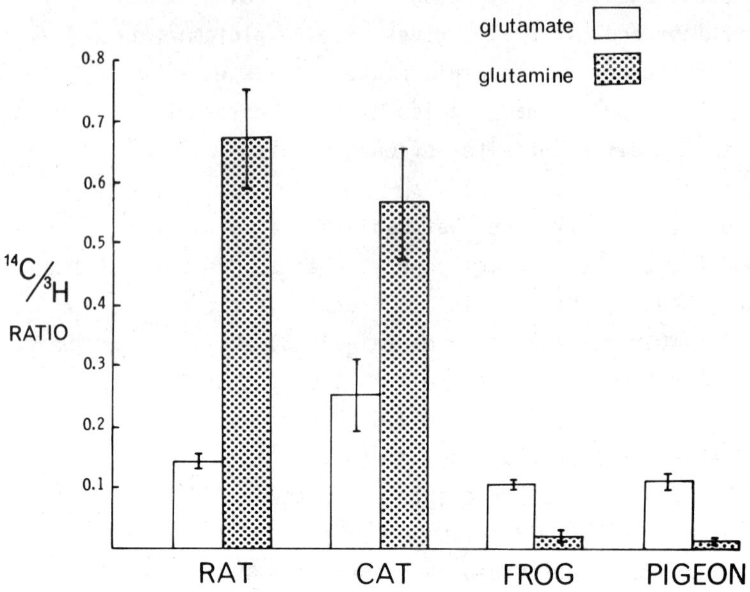

Fig. 5.5. The formation of glutamate and glutamine from ^{14}C GABA; in retinas from rat, cat, frog and pigeon. Experimental details have been given in the text. Following in vitro incubation with ^{14}C GABA for 60 min. retinal extracts were prepared and were reacted with ^{3}H dansyl chloride, to label the total free amino acid pool with tritium. Only the amino acids formed from ^{14}C GABA contain carbon 14. The final $^{14}C/^{3}H$ ratio for each amino acid is, therefore, a measure of its specific activity within the tissue. In rat and cat the specific activity of glutamine exceeds that of its precursor glutamate, whereas the reverse is true in frog and pigeon. (Voaden, Nathwani and Lake, unpublished observation).

has access to and is labeling a large percentage of the total tissue glutamate pool and that this is neuronal. Previous evidence has suggested that in cerebral cortex also large pools of glutamate are present in the neurones rather than the glia (Balázs et al., 1973).

We still have a great deal to learn about the various types of metabolic organization that can underly GABA utilisation in the central nervous system and the reasons for, and significance of neuronal as opposed to glial catabolic routes for GABA. It is to be hoped that studies on the retina will provide results relevant not only to the retina itself but also to less accessible areas of the central nervous system.

Functional aspects

In the preceding sections the species differences that exist in the metabolism of GABA within retinas have been emphasised. Possible species differences were not considered in the initial introduction to the evidence suggesting that GABA and glycine might be active in retinal neurotransmission. However, there are more specific observations which suggest that GABA has functional roles in both types of retinas.

Using the rat eye, Graham and Pong (1975) (see also Graham, 1974) have studied the effects of the intravitreal injection of GABA and its antagonists, picrotoxin and bicuculline, on the response of the retina to a light stimulus, and, in particular, on its adaptation to background lights of increasing intensity. They have found that GABA will mimic the effect of the background light and will decrease the sensitivity of the retina to the light stimulus. In contrast, the GABA antagonists have the reverse effect and increase sensitivity. In the experiments a point was reached above which gain sensitivity could not be affected. This was thought to coincide with the transition from scotopic to photopic vision. It may be, therefore, that in the rat retina the GABA system is specifically involved in second order adaptation mechanisms associated with the scotopic functioning of rod photoreceptor cells.

Effects of GABA and its antagonists on adaptation in the frog retina have not been reported. However, in this species, it is known that picrotoxin will change the waveform of the proximal negative response in a way that suggests blockade of a negative feedback process, perhaps at the bipolar-amacrine junction (Burkhardt, 1972). The PNR is an extracellular potential recorded from the inner neuronal layers of the retina and thought to reflect amacrine cell activity. Consistent with this it is normally seen as transient responses present at the on and/or off of a light stimulus. In the presence of picrotoxin, the waveform of the proximal negative response is altered and the response becomes slow and graded, and much more reminiscent of that seen in bipolars - the cells thought to drive amacrine interneurones. Strychnine is without effect. It seems therefore that, in the frog retina, GABA may be involved in the conversion of the visual impulse from the graded responses seen in the distal retina, to the more transient forms seen in proximal cells. It is not known whether the same is true in other species.

CONCLUDING REMARKS

GABA and glycine are present in retinas from a variety of species at levels similar to those found in brain. There is evidence that both are associated with amacrine cells and their synapses. GABA may be present also in horizontal cells, but species differences exist. Biochemical and preliminary neurophysiological studies suggest that both are neurotransmitters and more detailed neurophysiological information is now needed to establish the actual roles that the amino acids are playing in neurotransmission.

There are species differences in the ways that GABA is handled and whereas, in mammalian retinas, exogenously applied GABA can be taken up by glial cells, in some nonmammalian tissue (e.g. from frog, pigeon or chicken) it is taken up predominantly, if not solely, by neurones. When GABA goes into glia its carbon atoms enter a "small" glutamate pool active in the production of glutamine, whereas in neuronal metabolism it has access to a major percentage of the total tissue glutamate. In the latter case relatively less glutamine is produced.

In both types of retinas, overall metabolism appears organised in ways similar to other areas of the central nervous system. Retinas from various species are therefore, potential models for less accessible and possibly more complicated areas of the central nervous system where GABA may be taken up extensively by both neurones and glia.

ACKNOWLEDGEMENTS

I am indebted to my colleague Dr. John Marshall for preparing the autoradiographs included in this review, and to Dr. Norma Lake and Mrs. Bharti Nathwani for their help in the preparation of the manuscript.

My personal research has received financial support from the Medical Research Council, and the Wellcome Trust gave a travel grant which enabled me to participate in the symposium on transmitters in the visual process (Barcelona, September 1975). To both, I am grateful.

REFERENCES

Ames A., and Pollen D.A. (1969) Neurotransmission in central nervous tissue: a study of isolated rabbit retina. J. Neurophysiol. 32, 424-442

Balazs R., Patel A.J., and Richter D. (1973) Metabolic compartments in the brain: their properties and relation to morphological structures. In: Metabolic compartmentation in the brain. (R. Balazs and J.E. Cremer Eds.) pp 167-184. Macmillan London.

Berg C.J. van den (1973) A model of compartmentation in mouse brain based on glucose and acetate metabolism. In: Metabolic compartmentation in the brain. (R. Balazs and H.E. Cremer Eds.) pp 137-166. Macmillan London.

Bruun A., and Ehinger B. (1972) Uptake of the putative neurotransmitter, glycine, into the rabbit retina. Invest. Ophthal. 11, 191-198

Bruun A., and Ehinger B. (1974) Uptake of certain possible neurotransmitters into retinal neurones of some mammals. Exp. Eye Res. 19, 435-447

Burkhardt D.A. (1972) Effects of picrotoxin and strychnine upon electrical activity of the proximal retina. Brain Research, 43, 246-249

Cohen A.I., McDaniel M., and Orr H. (1973) Absolute levels of some free amino acids in normal and biologically fractionated retinas. Invest. Ophthal. 12, 686-693

Curtis D.R., and Johnston G.A.R. (1974) Amino acid transmitters in the mammalian central nervous system. Ergebn der Physiologie, 69, 98-188

Davis J.M., Himwich W.A., and Agrawal H.C. (1969) Some amino acids in the developing visual system. Dev. Psychobiol. 2, 34-39

Dowling J.E. (1970) Organization of vertebrate retinas. Invest. Ophthal. 9, 655-680

Dowling J.E., and Ripps H. (1973) Effect of magnesium on horizontal cell activity in the skate retina. Nature, 242, 101-103

Ehinger B., and Falck B. (1971) Autoradiography of some suspected neurotransmitter substances: GABA, glycine, glutamic acid, histamine, dopamine and L-dopa. Brain Research, 33, 157-172

Ehinger B., and Lindberg B. (1974) Light-evoked release of glycine from the retina. Nature, 251, 727-728

Goodchild M., and Neal M.J. (1973) The uptake of ^{3}H-gamma amino butyric acid by the retina. Brit. J. Pharmacol. 47, 529-542

Graham L.T., Baxter C.F., and Lolley R.N. (1970) In vivo influence of light or darkness on the GABA system in the retina of the frog (Rana pipiens). Brain Research, 20, 379-388

Graham L.T. jr. (1972) Intraretinal distribution of GABA content and GAD activity. Brain Research, 36, 476-479

Graham L.T. jr. (1974) Comparative aspects of neurotransmitters in the retina. In: The Eye, Volume 6 Comparative Physiology. (H. Davson and L.T. Graham jr. Eds.) pp 283-342. Academic Press, N.Y., London.

Graham L.T. jr., and Pong S.F. (1975) γ-aminobutyric acid (GABA) and sensitivity control in the scotopic mechanism of the rat retina. J. Physiol. (London) In press.

Hyde J.C., and Robinson N. (1974) Localisation of sites of GABA catabolism in the rat retina. Nature, 248, 432-433

Iversen L.L., and Neal M.J. (1968) The uptake of [^{3}H]GABA by slices of rat cerebral cortex. J. Neurochem. 15, 1141-1149

Johnston G.A.R., and Iversen L.L. (1971) Glycine uptake in the rat central nervous system slices and homogenates: Evidence for different uptake systems in spinal cord and cerebral cortex. J. Neurochem. 18, 1951-1961
Kelly J.S., and Krnjević K. (1969) The action of glycine on cortical neurones. Exp. Brain Res. 9, 155-163
Kennedy A.J., and Voaden M.J. (1974a) Free amino acids in the photoreceptor cells of the frog retina. J. Neurochem. 23, 1093-1095
Kennedy A.J., and Voaden M.J. (1974b) Distribution of free amino acids in the frog retina. Biochem. Soc. Trans. 2, 1256-1258
Kennedy A.J., and Voaden M.J. (1974c) Factors affecting the spontaneous release of [^{3}H]-γ-aminobutyric acid from the frog retina *in vitro*. J. Neurochem. 22, 63-71
Kennedy A.J., Voaden M.J., and Marshall J. (1974) Glutamate metabolism in the frog retina. Nature 252, 50-52
Krnjević K. (1974) Chemical nature of synaptic transmission in vertebrates. Physiol. Rev. 54, 418-540
Kuriyama K.E., Sisken B., Haber B., and Roberts E. (1968) The γ-aminobutyric acid system in rabbit retina. Brain Research 9, 165-168
Lam D.M.K., and Steinman L. (1971) The uptake of γ-^{3}H amino butyric acid in the goldfish retina. Proc. Nat. Acad. Sci. 68, 2777-2781
Lam D.M.K. (1972) The biosynthesis and content of gamma-aminobutyric acid in the goldfish retina. J. Cell Biol. 54, 225-231
Lam D.M.K. (1975) Biosynthesis of γ-aminobutyric acid by isolated axons of cone horizontal cells in the goldfish retina. Nature 254, 345-347
Macaione S., Ruggeri P., DeLuca F., and Tucci G. (1974) Free amino acids in developing rat retina. J. Neurochem. 22, 887-891
Marshall J., and Voaden M.J. (1974a) An investigation of the cells incorporating [^{3}H]GABA and [^{3}H]glycine in the isolated retina of the rat. Exp. Eye Res. 18, 367-370
Marshall J., and Voaden M.J. (1974b) A study of γ-(^{3}H) amino butyric acid and (^{3}H) glycine accumulation by the isolated pigeon retina utilizing scintillation radioautography. Biochem. Soc. Trans. 2, 268-270
Marshall J., and Voaden M.J. (1974c) An autoradiographic study of the cells accumulating [^{3}H]-γ-aminobutyric acid in the isolated retinas of pigeons and chickens. Invest. Ophthal. 13, 602-607
Marshall J., and Voaden M.J. (1975a) Further observations on the uptake of [^{3}H]glycine by the isolated retina of the frog. Exp. Eye Res. In press.
Marshall J., and Voaden M.J. (1975b) Autoradiographic identification of the cells accumulating ^{3}H-γ-aminobutyric acid in mammalian retinae: a species comparison. Vision Res. 14, 459-461
McIlwain H., and Bachelard H.S. (1971) Biochemistry of the central nervous system. 4th Edn. Churchill Livingstone, London
Minchin M.C.W., and Beart P.M. (1975) Compartmentation of amino acid metabolism in the rat posterior pituitary. J. Neurochem. 24, 881-884
Moore C.L., and Gruberg E.R. (1974) The distribution of succinic semialdehyde dehydrogenase in the brain and retina of the tiger salamander (Ambystoma tigrinum). Brain Research 67, 479-488
Murakami M., Ohtsu K., and Ohtsuka T. (1972) Effect of chemicals on receptors and horizontal cells in the retina. J. Physiol. (London) 227, 899-913
Neal M.J., and Iversen L.L. (1972) Autoradiographic localisation of ^{3}H-GABA in rat retina. Nature New Biol. 235, 217-218
Neal M.J., Peacock D.G., and White R.D. (1973) Kinetic analysis of amino acid uptake by the rat retina *in vitro*. Br. J. Pharmac. 47, 656-657 p.

Neal M.J. (1975) The uptake and release of γ-aminobutyric acid (GABA) by the retina. In: Transport phenomena in the nervous system; physiological and pathological aspects. Advances in Exp. Biol. and Med. A. Lajtha Ed. In press. Plenum Press. London & New York.

Nishi S., Minota S., and Karczmar A.G. (1974) Primary afferent neurones: the ionic mechanism of GABA mediated depolarization. Neuropharmacol. 13, 215-219

Pasantes-Morales H., Klethi J., Ledig M., and Mandel P. (1972) Free amino acids of chicken and rat retina. Brain Research, 41, 494-497

Pasantes-Morales H., Klethi J., Ledig M., and Mandel P. (1973) Influence of light and dark on the free amino acid pattern of the developing chick retina. Brain Research, 57, 59-65

Pasantes-Morales H., Klethi J., Urban P.F., and Mandel P. (1974) The effect of electrical stimulation, light and amino acids on the efflux of ^{35}S-taurine from the retina of domestic fowl. Exp. Brain Res. 19, 131-141

Starr M.S., and Voaden M.J. (1972) The uptake of ^{14}C-γ-aminobutyric acid by the isolated retina of the rat. Vision Research, 12, 549-559

Starr M.S. (1973) Effect of dark adaptation on the GABA system in retina. Brain Research, 59, 331-338

Starr M.S. (1974) Evidence for the compartmentation of glutamate metabolism in isolated rat retina. J. Neurochem. 23, 337-344

Starr M.S. (1975) Effect of light stimulation on the synthesis and release of GABA in rat and frog retinae. Brain Research, 100, 343-353

Stell W.K., Wagner H.G., and Wolbarsht M.L. (1970) Receptive field organization of ganglion cells in the retina of the smooth dogfish, Mustelus canis. Biol. Bull, 139, 437-438

Stell W.K. (1972) The morphological organization of the vertebrate retina. In: Handbook of sensory Physiology Vol/2: Physiology of photoreceptor organs. (M.G.F. Fuortes Ed.) pp 111-213

Toyoda J. (1973) Membrane resistance changes underlying the bipolar cell response in the carp retina. Vision Res. 13, 283-294

Toyoda J., Hashimoto H., and Ohtsu K. (1973) Bipolar-amacrine transmission in the carp retina. Vision Res. 13, 295-307

Voaden M.J., and Starr M.S. (1972) The efflux of radioactive GABA from rat retina in vitro. Vision Res. 12, 559-566

Voaden M.J. (1974) Light and the spontaneous efflux of radioactive glycine from the frog retina. Exp. Eye Res. 18, 467-475

Voaden M.J., Marshall J., and Murani N. (1974) The uptake of ^{3}H-γ-aminobutyric acid and ^{3}H glycine by the isolated retina of the frog. Brain Research, 67, 115-132

CHAPTER 6

ACETYLCHOLINE AS A RETINAL TRANSMITTER SUBSTANCE

Michael J. Neal

Department of Pharmacology
The School of Pharmacy
University of London
29/39 Brunswick Square
London, WCIN IAX

INTRODUCTION

It has been known for almost 50 years that the retina contains substantial amounts of acetylcholine (ACh). Also in some species, the choline acetyltransferase (ChAc) activity of the retina is extremely high. However, in spite of the demonstration many years ago that the retina possesses all the elements of the cholinergic system, the sites and function of the presumed cholinergic synapses are unknown.

The literature on ACh in the vertebrate retina has recently been comprehensively reviewed by Graham (1974). In this chapter, the information on the cholinergic system in the retina will be briefly reviewed and some recent experiments in our laboratory will be described.

ACETYLCHOLINE CONTENT

The most obvious criterion for a neurotransmitter is that the substance should be present in the tissue under consideration. ACh has been reported in the pig, dog, frog, chicken, ox and cow retina. The content of ACh (nmoles/g wet weight) in these retinae is in the range 5.7 (pig) to 33 (chicken and cow) (see Graham, 1974 for refs. and Fig. 6.1). The localisation of ACh within the retina is unknown. Invertebrate retinae seem to possess extremely high ACh contents. For example, the ACh content of the octopus retina is apparently 1300 nmoles ACh/g wet weight (Leo and Florey, 1966).

CHOLINE ACETYLTRANSFERASE

ChAc activity has been demonstrated in retinae of many different species (see Graham, 1974 for refs. and Fig. 6.1). Except in the pigeon, the optic nerve possesses little or no ChAc activity. The activity in the pigeon optic nerve may be related to the presence of centrifugal fibres in this species. In some species the retina possesses exceptionally high ChAc activity and Hebb (1955) pointed out that the chicken retina has the highest ChAc activity reported in vertebrate tissues. The ChAc activity of the retina shows a large species

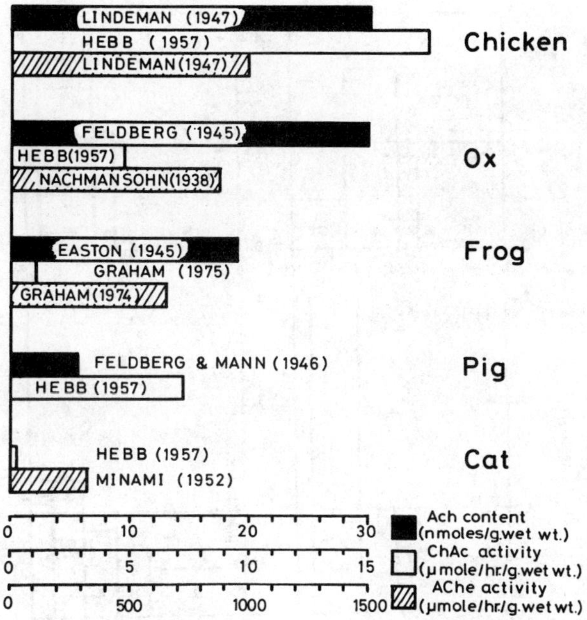

Fig. 6.1. Acetylcholine content, choline acetylase activity, and acetylcholine esterase activity in the retina of various species. Values taken from the recalculations of Graham (1974).

variation, the ratio between the highest activity (chicken retina) and the lowest activity (cat retina) being approximately 100 (Fig. 6.1). This large species difference must presumably reflect the relative importance of the cholinergic system in the retinae of different species but at present there does not seem to be any obvious correlation between ChAc activity and retinal structure or function. Cone retinae tend to have a higher ChAc activity, but the rat, which has a rod retina, also has a relatively high level of ChAc activity.

Intraretinal localisation of choline acetylase activity

There appears to have been only one study of the localisation of ChAc in the retina (Graham, Nurnberger and Pong, 1973). The results of these authors are illustrated in Fig. 6.2. In the pigeon, rat, and frog retina the ChAc activity is concentrated predominantly in the inner synaptic layer with smaller amounts of activity in the amacrine and ganglion cell layers. The receptor cell and

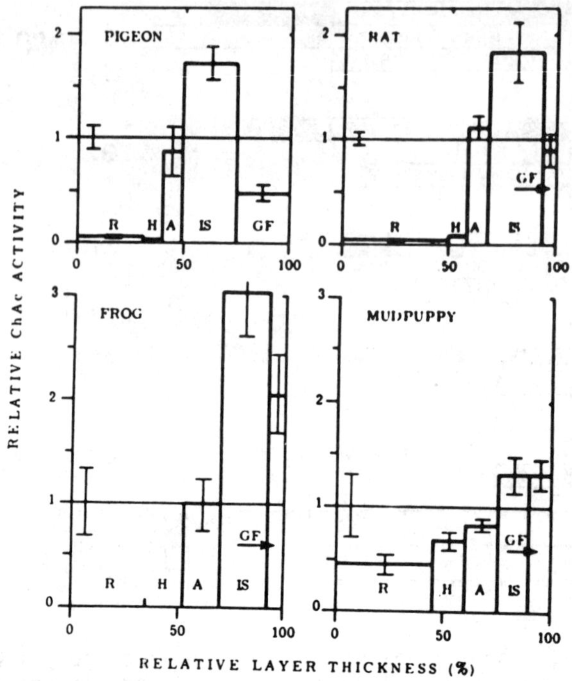

Fig. 6.2. Relative distribution of choline acetylase activity in the layers of several vertebrate retinae. The thickness of each layer relative to the whole retina is indicated and activities are compared with that obtained from samples across all layers. R = receptor, H = horizontal, A = amacrine, IS = inner synaptic, and GF = ganglion and nerve fibre layer. (Reproduced with permission from Graham et al., 1973).

horizontal cell layers in the pigeon and rat retinae show only relatively low ChAc activity and in the frog retina no activity at all is detected in these outer layers. These studies suggest that the cholinergic system is localised mainly in the inner retinal layers and that ACh is unlikely to be a photoreceptor or horizontal cell neurotransmitter, at least in the pigeon, rat and frog. However, the importance of considering species differences in retinal studies is reinforced by a recent study by Lam (1972) who found that isolated photoreceptor cells from the turtle retina could synthesise ACh but not GABA or dopamine. These results may suggest that ACh is a photoreceptor transmitter in the turtle, but they do not exclude the possibility of glutamate or aspartate being the major transmitter at the photoreceptor terminals. Lam et al. (1974) have also shown that cephalopod retinae are capable of synthesising ACh.

ACETYLCHOLINE ESTERASE

The activity of acetylcholine esterase in the retina is approximately 350 to 1000 μmoles/hr/g wet weight (Fig. 6.1) and in contrast to ChAc activity shows relatively little species variation (for refs. see Graham, 1974 and Fig. 6.1). Squid and octopus retinae possess very high activity (5,400 and 20,000 μmoles/hr/g wet weight respectively (Minami, 1952; Leo and Florey, 1966).

Intraretinal localisation

There appears to be only one report on the quantitative distribution of AChE in the retina. This report by Graham et al., (1973) indicates that in the pigeon retina the distribution of AChE activity parallels that of ChAc activity, i.e. it is concentrated predominantly in the inner synaptic layers. In contrast to the paucity of quantitative information, there have been numerous histochemical studies of AChE distribution. The interested reader should consult one of the many reviews on this subject (Nichols and Koelle, 1968; Reale et al., 1971; Stell, 1972). The histochemical studies of AChE distribution in the retina all agree that staining is concentrated in the inner synaptic layer and the variations of other structures which are quoted as staining for AChE seem to be the result of species variation and/or the techniques used. Koelle et al (1952) and Nichols and Koelle (1968) showed that in the cat, pigeon, squirrel, rabbit, and rat retina, specific AChE is localised only in cell bodies and processes of amacrine cells and concluded that these cells appear to be the major, if not the only, source of AChE in the inner synaptic layer.

EFFECTS OF ACETYLCHOLINE ON RETINAL NEURONES

There have been many studies which indicate that ACh and cholinergic drugs are capable of affecting neuronal activity in the retina. These studies suggest that ACh usually has an excitatory effect on retinal neurones. However, it should be remembered that although an effect of a putative transmitter is obviously necessary, such effects do not prove a substance is a transmitter.

Retinal ganglion cells are excited by ACh and eserine when these drugs are applied either iontophoretically (Noell and Lasansky, 1959) or by close arterial injection (Straschill, 1968). In contrast, ACh applied to the entire skate retina *in vitro* as a fine nebulised spray is without effect on the membrane potential of horizontal cells (Murakami, Ohtsu and Ohtsuka, 1972). There have been no reports on the effects of iontophoretically applied ACh on the membrane potential or membrane conductance of other types of retinal cell.

Ames and Pollen (1969) have studied the effect of several cholinergic drugs on the firing rate of ganglion cells of the superfused, isolated, rabbit retina. Eserine increases both spontaneous and evoked responses whilst curare at low concentrations depresses the activity of all cells. These results are consistent with ACh being a retinal transmitter and since hexamethonium also depresses ganglion cell firing and is much more effective than atropine, it would seem that the cholinergic receptors are nicotinic rather than muscarinic.

There have been several studies of the effects of cholinergic drugs on the electroretinogram but these have given contradictory results. Furthermore, the effects of drugs on such a complex response as the electroretinogram are very difficult to interpret in terms of transmitter action at specific synapses. The interested reader should refer to Graham (1974).

EFFECT OF LIGHT AND DARK ADAPTATION ON THE CHOLINERGIC SYSTEM

The ACh content of tissue is usually inversely related to neural activity. Thus, the results of Lange (1943) who found a tenfold increase of ACh in dark adapted retinae compared with those adapted to light are consistent with ACh being a retinal transmitter. Unfortunately, Lange's values for ACh are unbelievably high. Furthermore, Therman (1938) found no difference in ACh content with the adaptational state and Easton (1945) found only a very small increase in the ACh content of dark adapted retinae. This early work obviously needs repeating to clarify the important question of whether or not the adaptational state affects the ACh content of the retina. Graham et al. (1973) have recently shown that the ChAc activity in light and dark adapted retinae is not influenced by the state of adaptation.

It can be seen from the previous discussion that there is evidence to show that ACh satisfies some of the criteria for a transmitter role in the retina, i.e. it is present and the synthesising enzyme (ChAc) and the enzyme for its degradation (AChE) are also present. The identity of action criterion has not been adequately demonstrated, but ACh does have excitatory effects on retinal neurones. There have been no reports on the storage of ACh in the retina, i.e. whether or not it is present in nerve-endings and, more importantly perhaps, the release of ACh from the retina following photic stimulation has not been demonstrated.

We have recently started to study the subcellular distribution of the cholinergic system in the retina and also the synthesis and release of labelled ACh from retinae incubated with $[^3H]$choline. The results of these preliminary experiments will be described in the remainder of this paper.

CHOLINE UPTAKE IN THE RETINA

The uptake of choline into nerve terminals plays a vital role in cholinergic transmission. The uptake of choline into synaptosome preparations seems to be mediated by a transport system which possesses both a high and a low affinity component and there is evidence that in the brain it is the high affinity, sodium dependent system, that is associated with a high degree of ACh formation (Haga and Noda, 1973; Yamamura and Snyder, 1973). This high affinity choline uptake system is probably located in cholinergic nerve terminals since after lesions in the septum the ChAc activity of synaptosomes prepared from the hippocampus almost disappears and the ability of the synaptosomes to accumulate low concentrations of $[^3H]$choline is greatly reduced (Kuhar, Sethy, Roth and Aghajanian, 1973). However, not all high affinity choline transport processes are localized in cholinergic nerve endings, since it has been shown that the high affinity uptake process for choline in sympathetic ganglia is unaffected by denervation which causes a complete loss of cholinergic nerve terminals (Bowery and Neal, 1975). Because of the importance of choline transport processes in cholinergic systems, and because we wished to load the retina with labeled ACh, we have studied the uptake of $[^3H]$choline by the retina (Neal and Gilroy, 1975).

The uptake of N-[Me-^{3}H]choline (16.5 Ci/mmole, Radiochemical Centre, Amersham, Great Britain) has been studied using methods described in detail previously (Goodchild and Neal, 1973). Individual rat retinae or small pieces of rabbit retinae (approximately 10 mg wet weight) are given a preliminary incubation in 10 ml of Krebs bicarbonate medium at 37°C for 10 min. [^{3}H]Choline is then added to give a final concentration of 6.5 x 10^{-8}M (0.1 μCi/ml) and the incubations are continued for various times. The retinae are then briefly washed in medium and dissolved in 1.0 ml of Soluene 100 (Packard). The accumulated radioactivity is estimated by liquid scintillation counting after the addition of 10 ml butyl PBD (0.5%) in toluene. The results are calculated as the tissue-medium ratio (disint./min/g wet weight tissue : disint./min/ml medium). A tissue-medium ratio of 1.0 corresponds to 2.2 x 10^{3} disint./min being accumulated by a retina weighing 10 mg). The metabolism of [^{3}H]choline is studied by homogenising the tissue at the end of the incubation in ice-cold acid ethanol (95% ethanol, 0.2% acetic acid, 0.1 mM neostigmine and water) and subjecting the extract to electrophoresis.

Rat and rabbit retinae quickly accumulate radioactivity and after 50 min. incubation time, tissue: medium ratios of approximately 5 and 10 respectively are achieved (Fig. 6.3). The effect of different concentrations of choline on the uptake of [^{3}H]choline by the rat retina indicate that the uptake process is saturable. Kinetic analysis of the data suggest that the uptake process consists of two components: a low-affinity process (apparent Km = 100 μM) and a high-affinity process (Km = 2 μM). The kinetic parameters have been estimated by the method of least squares with arbitrary division of the data at 5 μM. They are similar to those reported recently for high- and low-affinity choline uptake processes in synaptosomes (Hage and Noda, 1973; Yamamura and Snyder, 1973) glial cell cultures (Massarelli, Sensenbrenner, Ebel and Mandel, 1974) and sympathetic ganglia (Bowery and Neal, 1975).

Both the high and low-affinity uptake processes for choline in the rat and rabbit retinae are temperature sensitive. At 0°C, the uptake of [^{3}H]choline (6 x 10^{-8}M or 1 mM) is reduced, tissue-medium ratios of less than one being achieved after 60 min. In contrast, the two processes show a difference in their requirements for external sodium ions. In the absence of sodium ions in the incubation medium, the uptake of [^{3}H]choline (1 mM) is unimpaired but the uptake of [^{3}H]choline (6 x 10^{-8}M) is reduced by 50%. We have not yet done any kinetic experiments on [^{3}H]choline uptake in the absence of sodium ions, but

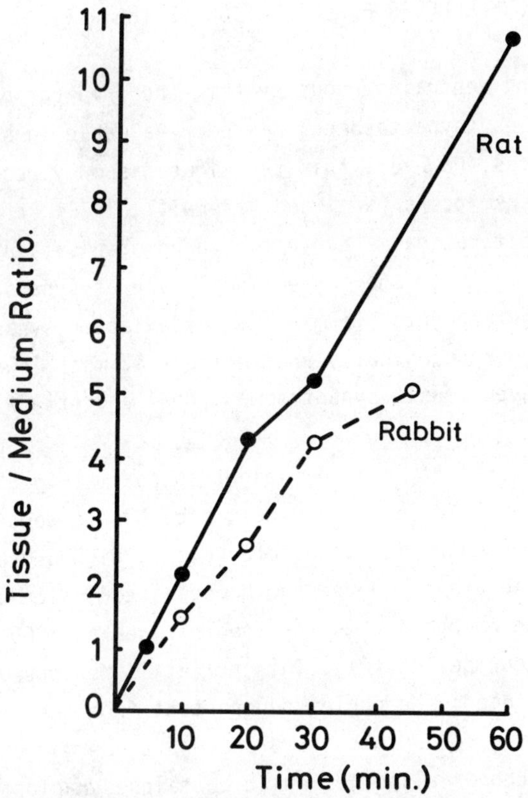

Fig. 6.3. Uptake of $[^3H]$choline by the rat and rabbit retina. Each point is the mean of at least 5 determinations and the S.E.M.'s were less than 8%.

calculations suggest that at 6 x 10^{-8}M choline the low affinity process would still contribute substantially to the choline uptake. This suggests that the high-affinity uptake process in the retina is highly sodium dependent. It seems likely, that the sodium dependent, high affinity uptake process for choline is associated with cholinergic nerve endings in the retina, because upon incubation of retinae with low concentrations of $[^3H]$choline (0.06 or 0.6 μM) a large proportion (50 to 60%) of the accumulated choline is converted to $[^3H]$ ACh. On the other hand, when retinae are incubated with high concentrations of $[^3H]$choline (60 μM) or a low concentration of choline (0.6 μM) in the absence of sodium ions, there is much less $[^3H]$ACh formation (20% and 3% respectively) (Neal and Gilroy, 1975).

SUBCELLULAR FRACTIONATION OF THE RETINA

In other areas of the central nervous system, the preparation of isolated nerve-ending particles (synaptosomes) has been valuable in studying central transmitter substances. However, this technique has only recently been applied to retinal transmitters (Neal and Atterwill, 1974; Atterwill and Neal, 1975). When the rabbit retina is subjected to homogenisation in sucrose, synaptosomes are formed from the conventional type of synapse in the retina and also from the photoreceptor terminals. These latter synaptosomes are easily identifiable morphologically and sediment at much lower centrifugation speeds than the "conventional" synaptosomes (Neal and Atterwill, 1974).

In the present study, rabbit retinae (weight approximately 500 mg) are incubated for 30 min. at 37°C in Krebs Ringer bicarbonate containing $[^{3}H]$ choline (6×10^{-8}M) i.e. a concentration associated with a high degree of $[^{3}H]$ ACh formation. The retinae are recovered and homogenised in ice cold 0.32 M sucrose (6% w/v). The homogenate is then centrifuged at 1000 g for 5 min. to produce a crude nuclear pellet (P1). This pellet is resuspended in 0.32 M sucrose and recentrifuged: the pooled supernatant from the two spins is then centrifuged at 17,000 g for 30 min. to produce a crude mitochondrial pellet (P2). The crude mitochondrial pellet which contains synaptosomes from the conventional type of retinal synapses (the photoreceptor terminals sediment largely in P1) is subfractionated by density centrifugation on a linear sucrose gradient (1.8 M to 0.4 M, total volume 8 ml). The P2 pellet is resuspended by gentle rehomogenisation in 0.32 M sucrose (7.0 ml/g original tissue), layered onto the gradient and centrifuged to apparent equilibrium at 100,000 g for 90 min. The gradient is then divided into 20-22 fractions by vacuum aspiration. Each fraction is assayed for radioactivity and for ChAc activity.

The distribution of radioactivity and ChAc on a continuous gradient is illustrated in Fig. 6.4. Approximately 80% of the radioactivity appears to be localised in particles which have an apparent medium equilibrium density equivalent to 1.25 M sucrose. More than 85% of the ChAc activity measured on the same gradients is also present in particles which have the same equilibrium density as those accumulating labelled choline. The "bound" radioactivity is reduced by 50% when the P2 pellet is exposed to hypo-osmotic con-

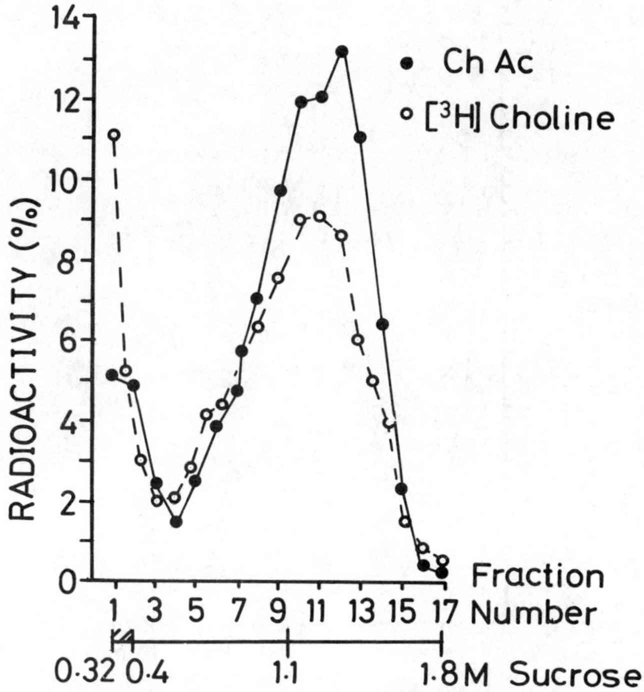

Fig. 6.4. Distribution of radioactivity and choline acetylase activity on linear sucrose density gradients. Retinae incubated with [^{3}H]choline were homogenised and a crude mitochondrial pellet obtained. The pellet was resuspended and layered onto the continuous gradient and centrifuged at 100,000 g for 90 min. Tritium and ChAc were determined on the same gradients and are expressed as % of the total activity on the gradient. The results illustrated represent a typical one of four experiments. (Atterwill and Neal, unpublished results).

ditions before centrifugation on the sucrose gradient (Fig. 6.5). Since ChAc is generally accepted as a synaptosomal marker, these results are consistent with the suggestion that at low concentrations, [^{3}H]choline is accumulated by cholinergic nerve-endings.

In order to obtain further information on the cholinergic system in the retina we have studied the distribution of ChAc, AChE and BuChE in primary fractions produced from rabbit retinae. The retinae are homogenised in 0.32 M sucrose and crude nuclear (P1), crude mitochondrial (P2) and supernatant

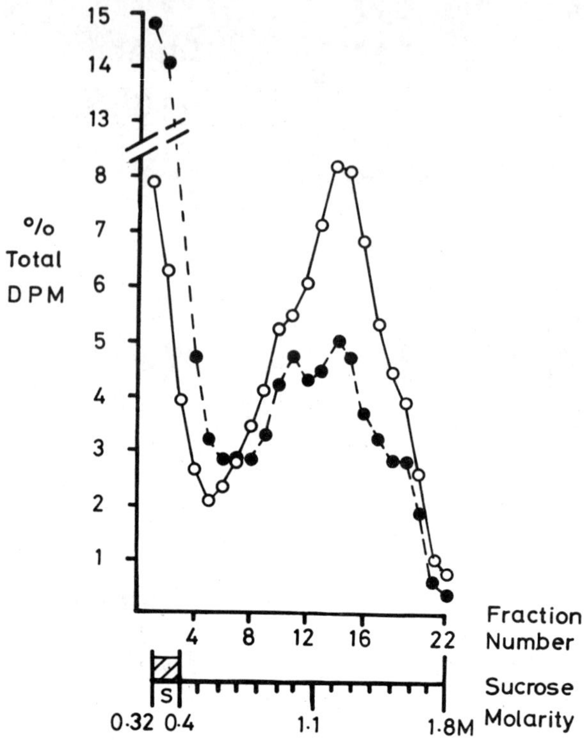

Fig. 6.5. Distribution of [^{14}C]choline after density gradient centrifugations of portions of crude mitochondrial fraction resuspended in isotonic (control O) or hypotonic (shocked ●) sucrose. The results shown represent a typical one of four experiments (Atterwill and Neal, unpublished results).

(SNT) fractions are obtained by differential centrifugation as described previously. The distribution of ChAc, AChE and BuChE in those fractions is shown in Fig. 6.6. ChAc activity is fairly evenly distributed between the three fractions, although in terms of relative specific activity (R.S.A.) the crude mitochondrial fraction (P2) possesses the highest activity. The relatively high proportion of ChAc in the SNT is probably due to the intraretinal nature of the cholinergic neurones. However, the origin of the considerable enzyme activity in P1 is not clear. It may be associated with the photoreceptor terminals or horizontal cell terminals which are sometimes attached to the photoreceptor terminals, but more likely perhaps, the ChAc activity may be

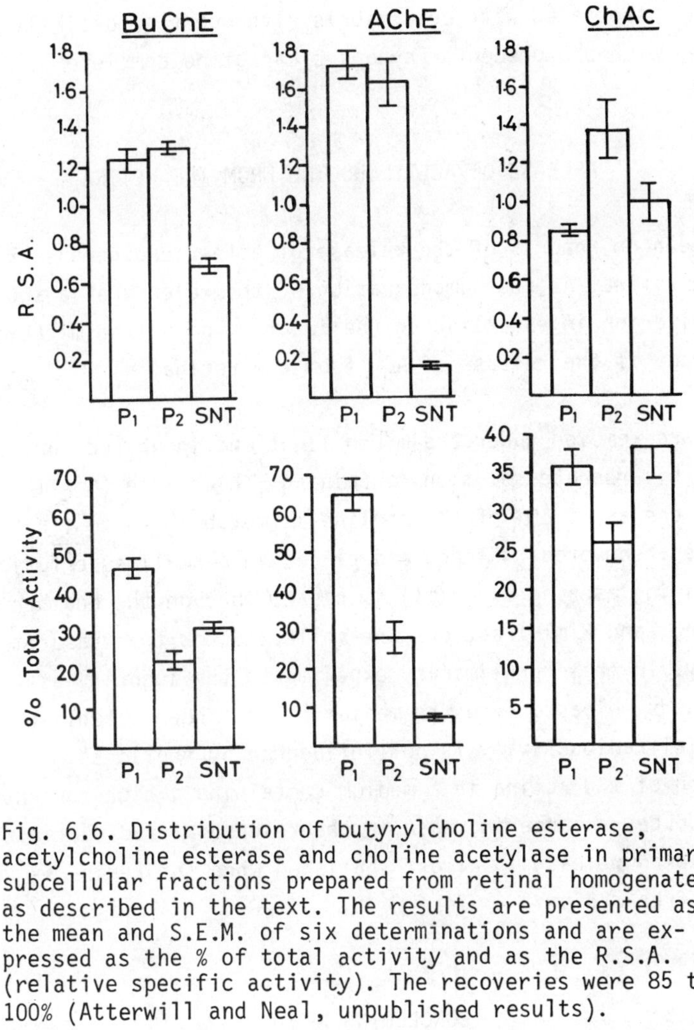

Fig. 6.6. Distribution of butyrylcholine esterase, acetylcholine esterase and choline acetylase in primary subcellular fractions prepared from retinal homogenates as described in the text. The results are presented as the mean and S.E.M. of six determinations and are expressed as the % of total activity and as the R.S.A. (relative specific activity). The recoveries were 85 to 100% (Atterwill and Neal, unpublished results).

associated with incompletely homogenised pieces of tissue.

AChE and BuChE have a similar subcellular distribution except that relatively more BuChE activity is found in the SNT fraction. Both enzymes are about equally distributed between P1 and P2. AChE and BuChE are usually considered to be bound to neuronal and glial cell membranes respectively. The presence of glial particles in P2 accounts for the presence of BuChE in this fraction and it is known that AChE is associated with the external membrane of synaptosomes which are presumably also present in P2. The activity of these enzymes in P1 is presumably associated with cell debris although the possibility that AChE is associated with photoreceptor synapses cannot be completely ruled out.

RELEASE OF ACETYLCHOLINE FROM THE RETINA

There have been no reports of the release of either endogenous or labelled ACh from the retina. As the demonstration of the release of a substance is an important criterion in establishing the identity of a transmitter, we have started a study of the release of ACh from the retina.

Rat retinae are removed under a dim red light and incubated for 30 min. in Krebs Ringer bicarbonate solution containing $[^3H]$choline (6×10^{-8}M). Under these conditions about 60% of $[^3H]$choline is metabolized to $[^3H]$ACh. Each retina is then recovered, washed, and placed in a small superfusion chamber. Medium containing eserine (1 mg/ml) is passed through the chamber at a rate of 0.5 ml/min., and 2 ml fractions are collected for the measurement of radioactivity. In these preliminary experiments the identity of the radioactive compounds released into the medium has not been established. The efflux of total radioactivity is not influenced by photic stimulation but depolarization of the retina in a medium containing a high concentration of potassium produces a large increase in the release of radioactivity (Fig. 6.7). This evoked release is almost abolished when the retina is superfused with calcium-free medium.

CONCLUDING REMARKS

The presence of ACh in the retina together with the sometimes exceptionally high levels of ChAc activity strongly suggest that cholinergic synapses occur in the retina. Other subsidiary findings such as the high affinity uptake for choline in the retina and the exceptionally high capacity for binding $[^{14}C]$ dimethyl-d-tubocurare (De Robertis and Fiszer, 1968) support this view. However, the identity of action and release criteria have not been established. The site and function of the presumed cholinergic synapses in the retina is unknown although several lines of investigation suggest that a population of amacrine cells may be cholinergic. This may perhaps be confirmed in the future

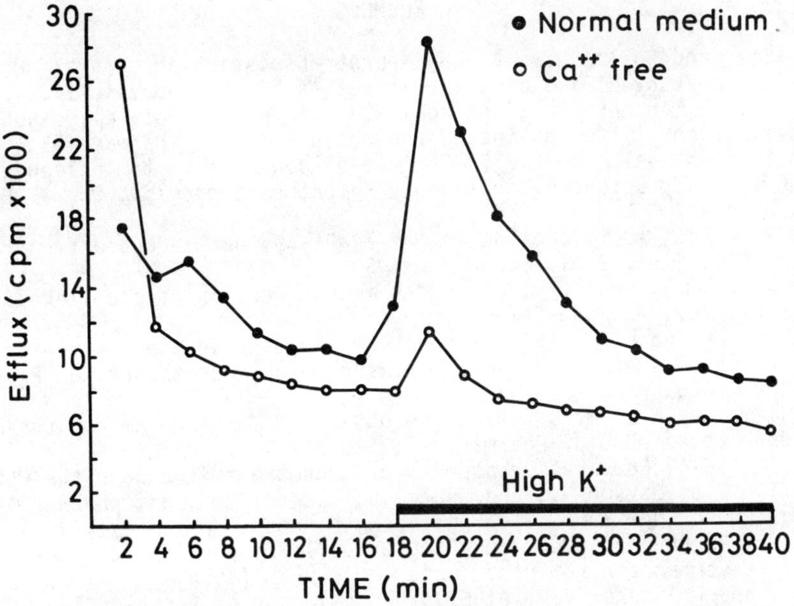

Fig. 6.7. Efflux of radioactivity from retinae previously incubated with [^{3}H]choline. The retinae are superfused in a small chamber with Krebs Ringer bicarbonate (●) or medium of identical composition except for the absence of calcium (O). After 18 min. the tissue is exposed to media containing potassium (40 mM). The results are the means of 6 determinations and the S.E.M. is less than 10%.

by the use of histochemical techniques to localise ChAc. The cholinoceptive cells are possibly ganglion cells and as the receptors appear to be nicotinic in character it may be possible to localise them by the use of labelled irreversible antagonists such as bungarotoxin. Until the sites of the cholinergic synapses are established, little progress can be made in understanding the role of ACh in the retina.

ACKNOWLEDGEMENT

This work was supported by the Medical Research Council.

REFERENCES

Ames A. III., and Pollen D.A. (1969) Neurotransmission in central nervous tissue: a study of isolated rabbit retina. J. Neurophysiol. 32, 424-442

Atterwill C.K., Mahoney Anne, and Neal M.J. (1975) The uptake and subcellular distribution of [^{3}H]choline by the retina. Br. J. Pharmac. 53, 447p

Bowery N.G., and Neal M.J. (1975) Failure of denervation to influence the high affinity uptake of choline by sympathetic ganglia. Br. J. Pharmac. 55, 278p

Easton D.M. (1945) Acetylcholine in the light-and dark-adapted frog retina. Proc. Soc. Expl. Biol. Med. 59, 31-33

Feldberg W. (1945) Present views on the mode of action of acetylcholine. Physiol. Rev. 25, 596-642

Feldberg W., and Mann T. (1946) Properties and distribution of the enzyme system which synthesizes acetylcholine in nervous tissue. J. Physiol. 104, 411-425

Goodchild M., and Neal M.J. (1973) The uptake of ^{3}H-gamma-aminobutyric acid by the retina. Br. J. Pharmac. 47, 529-542

Graham L.T. (1974) Comparative aspects of neurotransmitters in the retina, in: The Eye (Davson H., and Graham L.T. eds), Vol. VI, pp 283-342, Acad. Press, New York, San Francisco, London

Graham L.T., Nurnberger J.L., and Pong S.F. (1973) Choline acetylase activity in some vertebrate retinas. Quoted by Graham (1974)

Gray E.G., and Whittaker V.P. (1962) The isolation of nerve-endings from brain: an electron microscopic study of cell fragments derived by homogenization and centrifugation. J. Anat. (Lond). 96, 79-88

Haga T., and Noda H. (1973) Choline uptake systems of rat brain synaptosomes. Biochim. Biophys. Acta 291, 564-575

Hebb C.O. (1955) Cholineacetylase in mammalian and avian sensory systems. Quart. J. Exp. Physiol. 40, 176-186

Hebb C.O. (1957) The problem of identifying cholinergic neurones in the retina. Acta Physiol. Pharma. Neerl. 6, 621-631

Koelle G.B., Friedenwald J.S., Allen R.A., and Wolfand L. (1952) Localization of specific cholinesterase in ocular tissues of the cat. Am. J. Ophtal. 35, 1580-1584

Kuhar M.J., Sethy V.H., Roth R.H., and Aghajanian G.K. (1973) Choline: selective accumulation by central cholinergic neurons. J. Neurochem. 20, 581-593

Lam D.M.K. (1972) Biosynthesis of acetylcholine in turtle photoreceptors. Proc. Natn. Acad. Sci. 69, 1987-1991

Lam D.M.K., Wiesel T.N., and Kanekco A. (1974) Neurotransmitter synthesis in cephalopod retina. Brain Res. 82, 365-368

Lange V. (1943) Über das Vorkommon von Acetylcholine im hell-und dunkel-adaptieren Auge. Z. Physiol. Chem. 279, 73-76

Leo P.R., and Florey E. (1966) The distribution of acetylcholine and cholinesterase in the nervous system and in innervated organs of Octopus dofleini. Comp. Biochem. Physiol. 17, 509-522

Lindeman V.F. (1947) The cholinesterase and acetylcholine content of the chick retina with special references to functional activity as indicated by the pupillary constrictor reflex. Am. J. Physiol. 148, 40-44

Massarelli R., Sensenbrenner M., Ebel A., and Mandel P. (1974) Choline uptake in nerve cell cultures. Neurobiology 4, 293-300

Minami M. (1952) The location of cholinesterase in the retina. Acat. Soc. Ophthal. Jap. 56, 604-613

Murakami M., Ohtsu K., and Ohtsuka T. (1972) Effects of chemicals on receptors and horizontal cells in the retina. J. Physiol. 227, 899-913

Neal M.J., and Atterwill C.K. (1974) Isolation of photoreceptor and conventional nerve terminals by subcellular fractionation of rabbit retina. Nature 251, 331-333

Neal M.J., and Gilroy J. (1975) High affinity choline transport in the isolated retina. Brain Res. 93, 548-551

Nichols C.W., and Koelle G.B. (1968) Comparison of the localization of acetylcholinesterase and non-specific cholinesterase activities in mammalian and avian retinas. J. Comp. Neurol. 133, 1-15

Noell W.K., and Lasansky A. (1959) Effects of electrophoretically applied drugs and electrical currents on the ganglion cell of the retina. Fed. Proc. 18, 115

Reale E., Lucinano L., and Spitznas M. (1971) The fine structural localization of acetylcholinesterase activity in the retina and optic nerve of rabbit. J. Histochem. Cytochem. 19, 85-96

Robertis E. de, and Fiszer S. (1968) Distribution of acetylcholinesterase, proteolipids, and cholinergic receptor in cat brain. J. Pharm. Pharmacol. 20, 146-147

Stell W.K. (1972) The morphological organization of the vertebrate retina, in: Handbook of sensory physiology (Fuortes M.G.F. ed) Vol. VII, P2, pp 111-213. Springer-Verlag, Berlin

Straschill M. (1968) Action of drugs on single neurones in the cat's retina. Vision Res. 8, 35-47

Therman P.O. (1938) The neurophysiology of the retina in the light of chemical methods of modifying its excitability. Acta Soc. Sci. Fenn. Ser. (B2), 5-74

Yamamura H.I., and Snyder S.H. (1973) High affinity transport of choline into synaptosomes of rat brain. J. Neurochem. 21, 1355-1374

CHAPTER 7

BIOGENIC MONOAMINES AS TRANSMITTERS IN THE RETINA

B. Ehinger

Department of Ophthalmology
University of Lund
Lund
Sweden

INTRODUCTION

It is a well established concept that various chemicals act as neurotransmitters in both the central and peripheral nervous system, i.e. the presynaptic neuron releases a substance which will affect the postsynaptic membrane before it is inactivated by some mechanism. The motor end plate is presumably the best known example of such a chemical synapse. Structures with similar ultrastructure are abundant in the retina in all cell types and it is evident that all hitherto known retinal cell types operate with such synapses, even though other types of synapse may also be present (see chapter 1). As the detailed retinal ultrastructure is now being revealed and intracellular recordings have become possible in the retina, it is becoming important to establish the transmitter substances in the retina, and determine in which neurons they work.

Several criteria have to be fulfilled before a substance can be accepted as a neurotransmitter (see chapter 1, and also: Werman, 1972; Krnjević, 1974; or Curtis and Johnston, 1974). For no substance have all criteria been rigidly proven in the central nervous system, but for several there is sufficient evidence to consider them to be transmitters. The group of adrenergic substances belongs to this class.

A note on terminology is appropriate here. Only adrenaline can correctly be called an "adrenergic" transmitter, but dopamine and noradrenaline are also often included among adrenergic substances. This is the meaning of the term "adrenergic" in many histochemical papers by different authors cited here, and the reader should remember this when returning to these papers. However, all three substances are catecholamines, and "catecholamine containing" or "catecholaminergic" are, therefore, more appropriate terms. 5-Hydroxytryptamine is at times also included among the "adrenergic" substances, presumably because like noradrenaline, dopamine and adrenaline it is demonstrable with the Falck-Hillarp histofluorescence procedure. In this case the term "tryptaminergic" or "serotoninergic" or "indolamine containing" is preferable. When both catecholamines and indolamines are being discussed, the term "biogenic monoamines" seems most appropriate.

HISTOCHEMICAL DEMONSTRATION OF CATECHOLAMINES AND INDOLAMINES

Formaldehyde reacts with the amines noradrenaline, dopamine, adrenaline and 5-hydroxytryptamine under the formation of highly fluorescent compounds: isoquinolines from noradrenaline, dopamine and adrenaline; carbolines from 5-hydroxytryptamine (Falck, 1962; Falck, Hillarp, Thieme and Torp, 1962; Björklund et al., 1973). For optimal yield of fluorescence, the reaction is dependent on a low but critical humidity and the tissues must therefore usually be freeze-dried and processed under low, controlled humidity. Also, the tissue proteins play an important catalytic role in the reaction. The procedure is technically somewhat demanding, but detailed descriptions of it have been published (Falck and Owman, 1965; Corrodi and Johnsson, 1967; Björklund et al., 1972; Eränkö, 1967; Björklund and Falck, 1973).

5-Hydroxytryptamine gives a yellow fluorescence, which in the microscope is readily distinguishable from the green (or blue, depending on the filter settings in the microscope) colour of the catecholamine fluorescence. Under ordinary circumstances, the fluorescence caused by noradrenaline cannot be readily distinguished from that of dopamine and adrenaline. However, by microspectrofluorometry it is possible to distinguish dopamine and noradrenaline (Björklund, Ehinger and Falck, 1968 and 1972). Adrenaline does not readily form fluorophores with formaldehyde, and to some extent this fact can be used to identify structures containing it (Falck, Häggendal and Owman, 1963). Various pharmacological pretreatments have also been used in order to make visible only neurons with either of the three transmitters (see e.g. Carlsson, Dahlström, Fuxe and Hillarp, 1965; Carlsson, Fuxe, Hamberger and Lindquist, 1966; Carlsson, Lindquist, Fuxe and Hökfelt, 1966; Ehinger and Falck, 1969).

Not only noradrenaline, dopamine, adrenaline and 5-hydroxytryptamine give strongly fluorescent products when reacting with formaldehyde, but also a number of other related substances (Björklund, Falck and Owman, 1972; Björklund and Falck, 1973). These are, however, of only limited interest when discussing neurotransmitters. It may be noted here that acetylcholine, histamine, melatonin and any of the biogenic amino acids are not demonstrable in this way.

HISTOCHEMISTRY OF CATECHOLAMINE CONTAINING NEURONS IN THE RETINA

Unlike the silver staining techniques, the Falck-Hillarp procedure will show all neurons containing a catecholamine. It also demonstrates the processes, which form a densely intertwined network in which it is impossible to trace individual fibres. It is therefore usually not possible to characterize individual cells from the distribution of the processes, or even to state in more than a very general fashion the origin of the terminals found in a particular layer. The cell bodies and their characteristics will therefore be treated separately from the terminals.

A) Cell bodies

Catecholamine containing cell bodies appear in all species in the innermost cell row of the inner nuclear layer, among the amacrine cells (Fig. 7.1-7). They represent 5 to 10 percent of the total number of cell bodies in this layer. Much less frequently, catecholamine containing cells bodies appear among the ganglion cells (Fig. 7.7) and, even less frequently, in the middle of the inner plexiform layer. The three types have been named junctional cells, alloganglion cells and eremite cells, respectively. They have been observed in all species so far examined:

several species of fish (Fig. 7.1), Ehinger, Falck and Laties, 1969;
frogs and toads (Fig. 7.2);
gecko, Scheie and Laties, 1971;
lizards (Lacerta viridis), Ehinger unpublished;
mudpuppy (Necturus maculosus), Laties personal communication, Ehinger unpublished;
rat (Fig. 7.3), Malmfors, 1963; Ehinger, 1966; Nichols, Jacobowitz and Hottenstein, 1967;
mouse, Ehinger and Falck, 1969;
flying fox (Pteropus giganteus), Ehinger, 1973;
guinea-pig, Ehinger, 1966; Nichols, Jacobowitz and Hottenstein, 1967;
rabbit (Fig. 7.4), Häggendal and Malmfors, 1963 and 1965; Ehinger, 1966; Laties and Jacobowitz, 1966; Nichols, Jacobowitz and Hottenstein, 1967;
cat, Laties and Jacobowitz, 1966; Ehinger and Falck, 1969;
dog, Sano, Yoshikawa and Konishi, 1968;

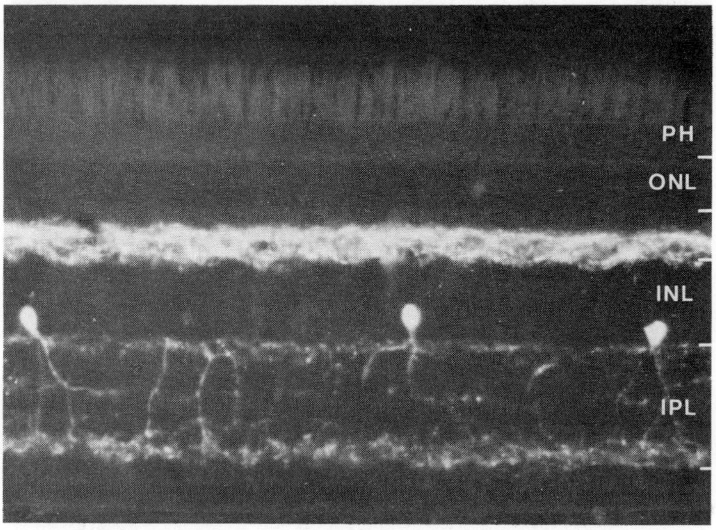

Fig. 7.1. Perch retina. There are three fluorescent perikarya in the innermost cell row of the inner nuclear layer (INL). They send their processes to three not very well defined sublayers of the inner plexiform layer (IPL). There is also a dense network of terminals around the horizontal cells (arrows). Very fine fibres connect the inner and outer plexiform layers, but these fibres are too weakly fluorescent to photograph well. Ph, photoreceptors; ONL, outer nuclear layer; G, ganglion cell layer. X 240.

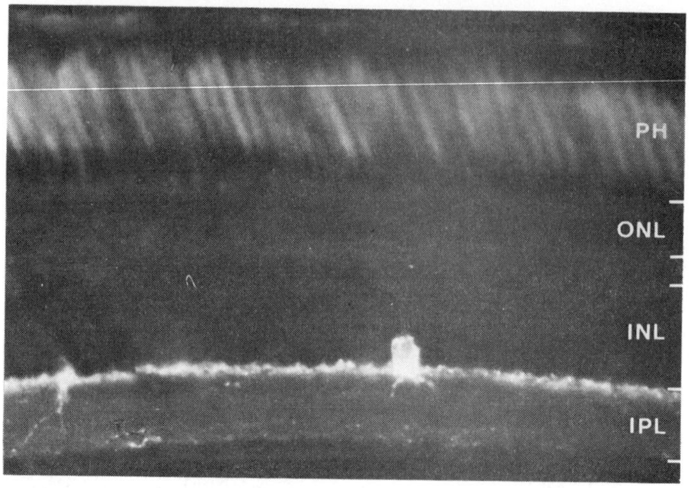

Fig. 7.2. Frog retina (Rana pipiens). There is one complete fluorescent perikaryon and parts of another in the innermost part of the inner nuclear layer. Both send processes to one well-defined sublayer at the border between the inner nuclear and inner plexiform layers, and another, much less defined sublayer in the innermost part of the inner plexiform layer. Designation of layers as in Fig. 7.1. X 230.

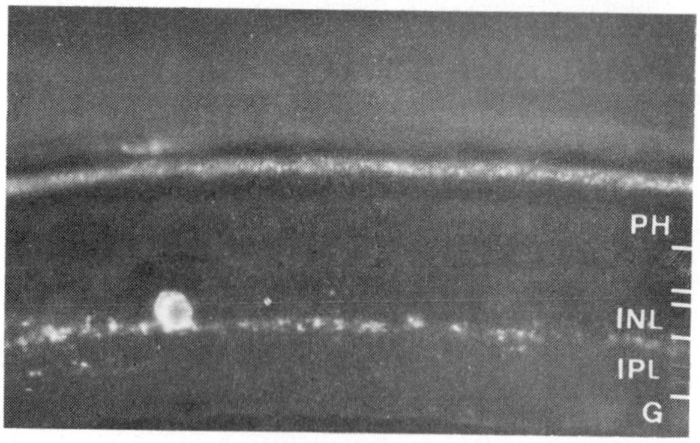

Fig. 7.3. Rat retina. There is one fluorescent perikaryon in the innermost part of the inner nuclear layer and one sublayer of fluorescent terminals at the border between the inner nuclear and inner plexiform layers. In addition, there are some few fluorescent terminals in the middle of the inner plexiform layer. Designation of layers as in Fig. 7.1. X 245.

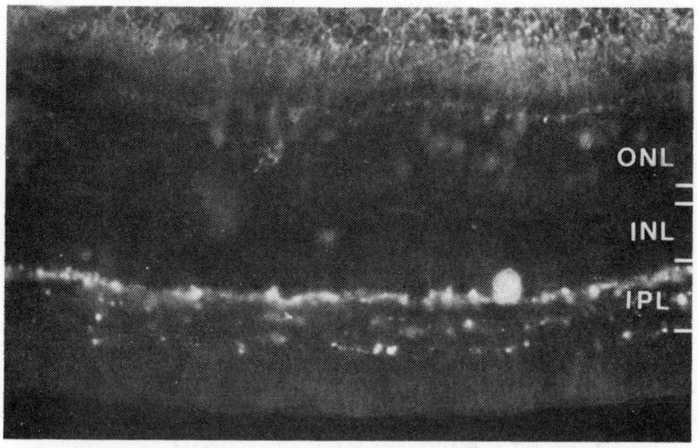

Fig. 7.4. Rabbit retina. There is one fluorescent perikaryon in the innermost part of the inner nuclear layer and three sublayers of fluorescent terminals in the inner plexiform layer. Designation of layers as in Fig. 7.1. X 300.

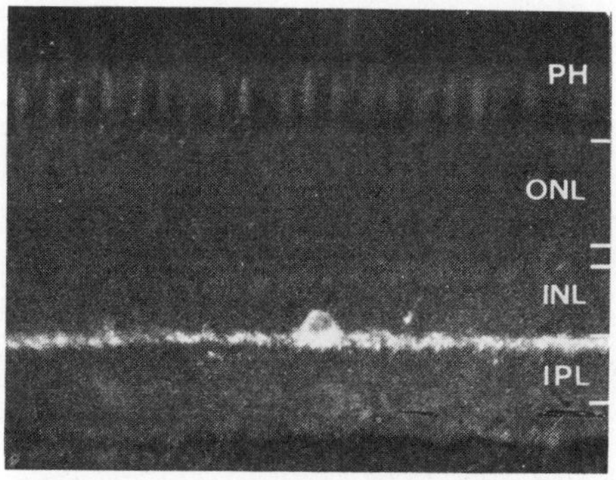

Fig. 7.5. Monkey (<u>Cynomolgus irus</u>)retina. There is one fluorescent perikaryon in the innermost part of the inner nuclear layer and one sublayer of fluorescent terminals at the border between the inner nuclear and inner plexiform layers. Note the difference between this retina and that of the Cebus monkey (Fig. 7.6). Designation of layers as in Fig. 7.1. X 300.

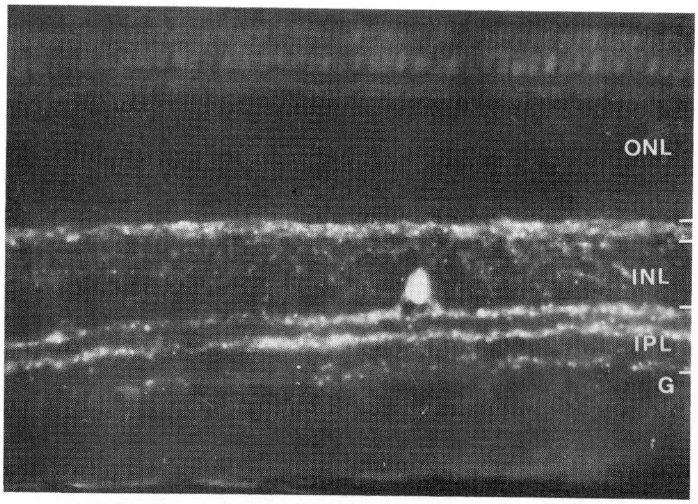

Fig. 7.6. Monkey (Cebus capucinus) retina. In addition to the fluorescent perikaryon in the innermost part of the inner nuclear layer there are three sublayers of terminals in the inner plexiform layer and a plexus of terminals in the inner nuclear layer, reaching out as far as the outer plexiform layer. Note the difference between this retina and that of the Cynomolgus retina (Fig. 7.5). Designation of layers as in Fig. 7.1. X 320.

macaque monkeys (Fig. 7.5), Ehinger, 1966; Laties and Jacobowitz, 1967;
vervet monkeys (Cercopithecus ethiops), Laties and Jacobowitz, 1967; Ehinger unpublished;
patas monkeys and baboons, Ehinger unpublished;
Cebus (Fig. 7.6), squirrel, owl and marmoset monkeys, Ehinger and Falck, 1969; Laties, personal communication;
humans, Ehinger, 1966; Laties, personal communication.
They have not been observed in birds, where only the junctional cells have been found (chicken, duck and pigeon, Ehinger, 1967).

A fourth type of cell body has been seen in Cebus monkeys, situated in the middle of the inner nuclear layer (Ehinger and Falck, 1969), which has been called the pleomorph cell (Fig. 7.7). Two subgroups of junctional cells were seen in some New World monkeys, one larger and one smaller (Ehinger and Falck, 1969).

Studies after severing or crushing the optic nerve have shown that the retinal catecholamine containing neurons are all wholly intraretinal. There are no catecholamine containing axons among the optic nerve fibres, either centrifugal or centripetal, in rat, cat, rabbit, and squirrel monkey (Ehinger and Falck, 1969).

B) Terminals

1) Mammals

Terminals occur in the inner plexiform layer in all species. Usually the terminals occur in three more or less well-defined sublayers: one at the outer border of the inner plexiform layer, one in the middle of it, and one at its inner border close to the ganglion cells. In all mammals the outermost layer is best developed, and in mouse, rat, cat, vervet monkey, cynomolgus monkey, macaque monkey, patas monkey and humans (caucasians) this is the only layer except for occasional branches elsewhere. The references to the papers on the various species can be found in the previous section on cell bodies.

All catecholamine containing cell bodies, irrespective of their position, send their branches to the outermost sublayer. In rabbit (Fig. 7.4), dog and Cebus

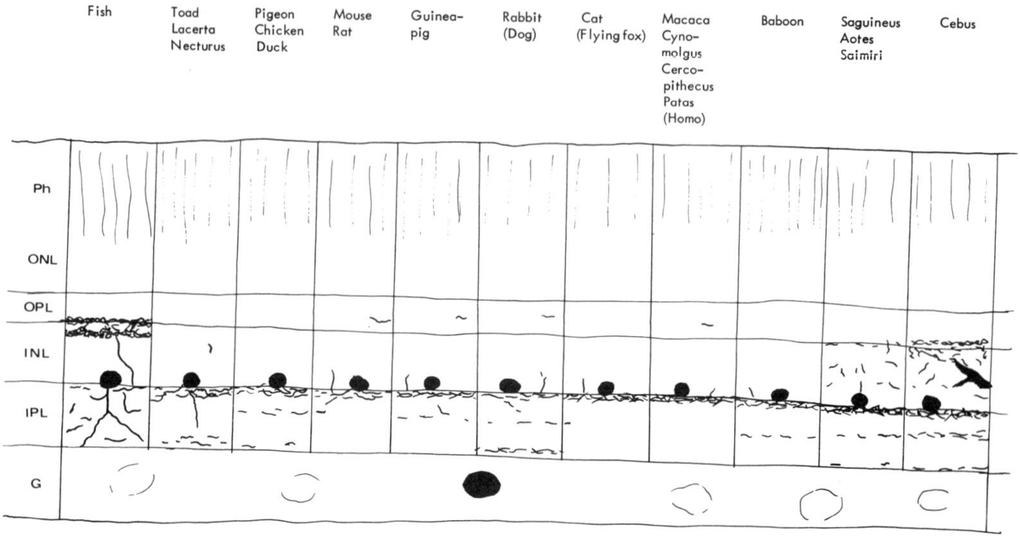

Fig. 7.7. Schematic drawing of the distribution of catecholamine containing neurons in the retina of different species. The lines separating the species have not been extended to the ganglion cell layer, because here no species differences have been observed, except in birds where there are no fluorescent cells in this layer. The parentheses around some of the species names indicate that these species show certain additional features which have not been included in the figure. For these the original papers should be consulted.

monkey (Fig. 7.6) all three sublayers are present (Fig. 7.7), the middle being the least developed in rabbits, the inner sublayer in the Cebus monkey. The three layers receive fibres from either junctional cells, alloganglion cells or eremite cells. Two sublayers, the outer and the middle, have been seen in guinea-pig, baboon (Papio papio) and some New World monkeys (Saimiri sciurea, Saguineus oedipus, Aotes trivirgatus) (Fig. 7.7).

In all the New World monkeys mentioned above there is also a plexus of catecholamine containing fibres throughout the inner nuclear layer (Laties and Jacobowitz, 1966; Ehinger and Falck, 1969; Dowling and Ehinger, 1975; Dowling et al., 1975). It is best developed in the Cebus (Fig. 7.6), where the fibres form a sublayer in the outer plexiform layer. (For a further discussion of these fibres, see below under Electron microscopy.) These fibres originate from the junctional cells, and in Cebus also from the catecholamine containing pleomorph cells, which have been observed in this species only (see above). In no other of the mammals studied so far, significant numbers of comparable catecholamine containing fibres have been seen, despite careful search. At times a few fibres can be seen to form baskets of synaptic character around a non-catecholaminergic amacrine cell body. Rarely an isolated catecholamine containing branch can be seen winding through the inner nuclear layer towards and even reaching the outer plexiform layer, but never in amounts comparable to what is seen in Cebus or squirrel monkey. However, as described below, numerous such fibres occur in teleost fish.

2) Birds.
In pigeon, chicken and duck, catecholamine containing terminals occur in three sublayers of the inner plexiform layer, one at its outer border, one in its middle and one at its inner border (Ehinger, 1967). The outermost layer is most developed. The position of the layers (Fig. 7.7) is thus comparable to that of some mammals (such as rabbit), but the relative number of fibres in different sublayers varies.

3) In reptiles and amphibians (gecko: Gecko gecko, toad: Rana pipiens, lizard: Lacerta viridis, mudpuppy: Necturus maculosus) the sublayering in the inner plexiform is somewhat less noticeable than in mammals and birds, and terminals occur throughout the layer. Two sublayers are nevertheless often seen (Fig. 7.2), the best developed being at the outer border, and the other at the inner border. There are catecholamine containing terminals around some few cell bodies among the amacrines, and there is an occasional branch running towards the outer plexiform layer.

4) In teleost fish (Fig. 7.1), the terminals of the inner plexiform layer are distributed throughout it, with only poorly defined sublayers. In addition, there are fine preterminal twigs issuing outwards through the inner nuclear layer, forming a dense plexus of terminals around the horizontal cells. The system resembles that seen in New World monkeys, but the density of terminals around the horizontals is much higher in fish than in monkeys. It will be described in more detail below, in connexion with electron microscopy.

EVOLUTIONARY ASPECTS

The distribution of catecholamine containing terminals in various species is summarized in Fig. 7.7. It is apparent that there is no simple evolutionary pattern. It seems that in going from fish via reptiles and amphibians to birds, the fibres of the inner plexiform layer become simplified and more strictly organized. This is in keeping with the assumption (Dowling, 1968) that during evolution the signal processing in the retina has been simplified and the more qualified stimulus analysis has been progressively taken over by higher centres. However, among mammals this pattern of progressively increasing simplicity is not apparent. Complex fibre patterns appear in rabbit, dog and some New World monkeys, simple patterns occur in mouse, rat, cat, some Old World monkeys and humans. However, it would seem that the human retina has more in common with some Old World monkeys than with those of the New World.

It is of considerable interest to note the plexus of catecholamine containing fibres in the inner nuclear layer and outer plexiform layer. This plexus occurs in teleost fish (Fig. 7.1) and some New World monkeys (Fig. 7.6), as is apparent from the findings of Laties and Jacobowitz (1966), Ehinger, Falck and Laties (1969), and Ehinger and Falck (1969). Electron microscopy (see below) has strongly suggested that these fibres mediate a centrifugal intraretinal impulse flow. Silver stainings suggest that these fibres occur also in cat, rabbit and rhesus monkey (Boycott et al., 1975), but fluorescence microscopy fails to show any such neurons in these species. Knowing that the main catecholamine transmitter in the retina is dopamine (see below) and also that substances fairly closely related to dopamine, such as octopamine or tyramine, are invisible in the fluorescence microscope, one might conjecture that the transmitter of the interplexiform cells in sub-primate mammals might be such a dopamine derivative. If so, they should (by analogy with catecholaminergic neurons) accumulate not only their actual transmitter, but also dopamine, noradrenaline or other related substances. Experiments designed to show this (Ehinger, unpublished) have given negative results. This suggests that the transmitter of the interplexiform cells of sub-primate mammals is not a substance closely related to dopamine.

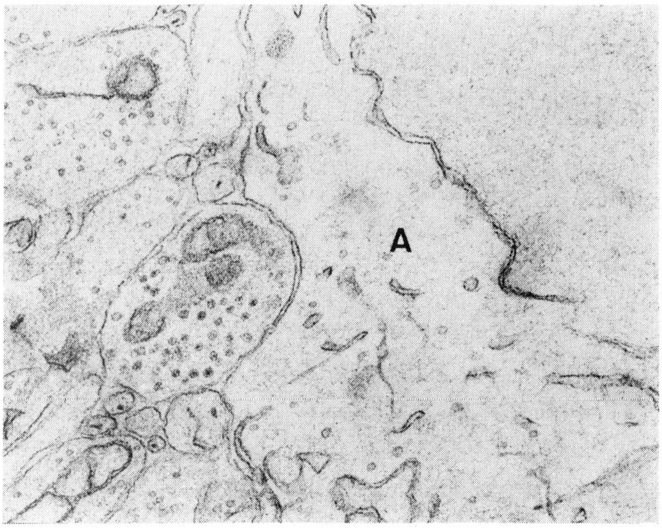

Fig. 7.8. Cat retina, taken four hours after intravitreal injection of 100 μg α-methyldopamine. One of the axon profiles contains numerous synaptic vesicles with a small dense core. A is an ordinary amacrine cell. Permanganate fixation. No synaptic specializations are observed with this type of fixation. X 25600.

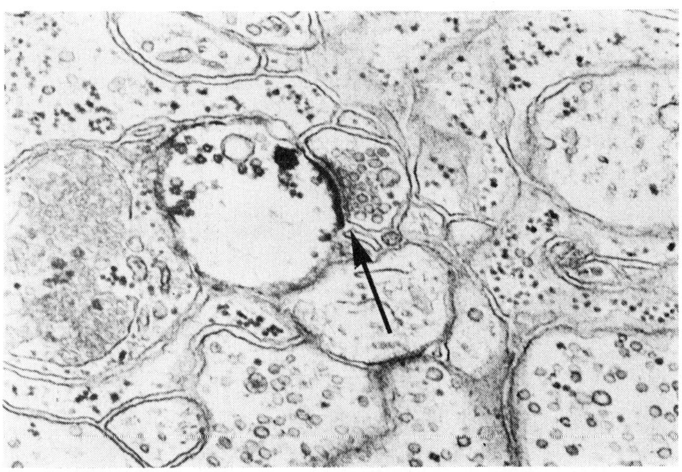

Fig. 7.9. Rabbit retina, taken four hours after intravitreal injection of 50 μg 5,6-dihydroxytryptamine. There is one axon profile showing swelling, increased membrane density, and some small vesicles with increased electron density. An ordinary amacrine cell process is making a conventional synapse onto the altered process (arrow). Osmium tetroxyde fixation. X 32800.

ELECTRON MICROSCOPY OF CATECHOLAMINERGIC RETINAL NEURONS

It is now possible to classify electron microscopically the various processes and their synapses in the plexiform layers. It is of obvious interest to try to identify the transmitter of individual terminals, and to analyze their synaptic connexions. Some years ago it was suggested that the so-called dense cored synaptic vesicles are typical the catecholamine containing neurons. Large (800-1000 Å) vesicles of this type also occur in retinal axon profiles (Pellegrino de Iraldi and Etcheverry, 1967). However, the distribution of these profiles does not agree very well with that of the catecholamine containing fibres seen with the fluorescence microscope. Later, it has been shown that the large dense cored vesicles are not specific for catecholaminergic neurons, but only the small type (diameter 300-500 Å). The latter are visible only in dopamine containing CNS neurons after prior loading with a catecholamine (such as α-methyldopamine, which is resistant to degradation by monoamine oxidase), followed by fixation in potassium permanganate (Hökfelt, 1967 and 1968; Hökfelt and Jonsson, 1968). This is also the case in the retina (Fig. 7.8), but with this type of fixation identification of synapses is unfortunately impossible.

Catecholaminergic neurons will actively accumulate not only their transmitter but also other related substances. This fact can be utilized to tag such neurons in various ways. It has been observed that 5,6-dihydroxytryptamine is accumulated by the retinal catecholamine containing neurons, and will produce typical changes in these neurons, making them readily visible in the electron microscope (Dowling and Ehinger, 1975). In short, the changes consist of the appearance of small (about 500 Å) dense cored synaptic vesicles, increased electron density of the cytoplasm and increased electron density of mitochondrial and cell membranes (Fig. 7.9). With this procedure, the synaptic contacts of the remarkable catecholamine containing plexus in the inner nuclear and outer plexiform layers of goldfish and Cebus monkeys have been analyzed (Dowling and Ehinger, 1975). There are no morphological signs of an input into these neurons other than in the inner plexiform layer, but numerous examples of synapses onto both horizontal cells and bipolar cells (in both plexiform layers) have been found. These processes must therefore represent a

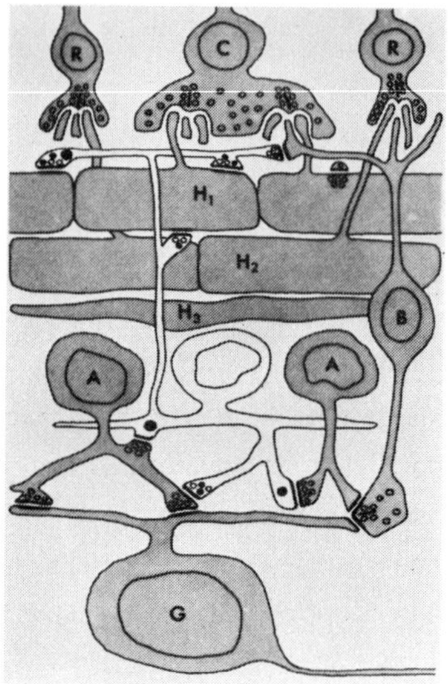

Fig. 7.10. A summary diagram of the synaptic connections of the interplexiform cells of the goldfish retina. The input to these neurons is in the inner plexiform layer via conventional synapses of amacrine cells (A). The interplexiform cells have been observed to make conventional synapses onto amacrine cell processes in the inner plexiform layer, but they never contact the ganglion cells (G) or their dendrites. In the outer plexiform layer, the processes of the interplexiform cells make synapses on the perikarya of the external horizontal cells (H_1) and onto bipolar cell (B) dendrites. The interplexiform cell processes are never observed as postsynaptic elements in the outer plexiform layer at either rod (R) or cone (C) receptor terminal synapses or at the occasional external horizontal cell synapse. (From Dowling and Ehinger, 1975).

special type of cell, named the interplexiform neuron, transmitting information centrifugally from the inner plexiform layer to the outer plexiform layer (Fig. 7.10). The interplexiform neuron processes come fairly close to the cone pedicles, but no actual contacts suggesting synapses have been seen. As best seen in fluorescence micrographs (Fig. 7.1), there is a significant number of such neurons, indicating that they have more than a marginal role in retinal function.

IDENTITY OF THE CATECHOLAMINES IN THE RETINA

As noted above, noradrenaline and dopamine cannot be directly distinguished with the Falck and Hillarp method, unless special pharmacological or microspectrofluorometric procedures are employed. Thus the fluorescent neurons observed in routine fluorescence microscopy may contain either or both of these substances. Adrenaline also gives rise to a fluorescence that is difficult to distinguish from that of dopamine or noradrenaline, but a special procedure is necessary to elicit it. Specific fluorescence attributable to adrenaline has not been observed in the retina, but it cannot be excluded that a minor cell population could contain it.

Pharmacologically, noradrenaline containing neurons can be selectively depleted, and in such experiments the retinal neurons remain without observable change, thus suggesting they contain dopamine. Chemically, dopamine has been shown to be the dominating catecholamine, with a concentration of 0.1-0.2 μg/g wet weight in rabbits or 10-15 μg per retina (Häggendal and Malmfors, 1965; Nichols, Jacobowitz and Hottenstein, 1967). Drujan et al. (1965) has reported figures around 1-2 μg/g. Some noradrenaline has also been reported, but it was felt that this represents a contamination by choroid and other non-retinal tissues. On the other hand, pharmacological experiments aimed at depressing the dopamine fluorescence while retaining that from noradrenaline show a few fluorescent cell bodies and terminals, suggesting that these cells may contain noradrenaline (Ehinger and Falck, 1969). Adrenaline is reported in significant amounts in the frog and in lower amounts in the toad (Drujan, Diáz Borges and Alvarez, 1965; Drujan and Diáz Borges, 1968).

Dopamine and noradrenaline can be histochemically distinguished by microspectrofluorometry. Only dopamine has been detected in the species so far investigated: rat, rabbit, cynomolgus and squirrel monkey, perch (Ehinger, unpublished). Clearly, this does not exclude that there may be a small population of noradrenaline containing cells hidden among the dopaminergic ones. Further, with this method it is difficult to observe small amounts of noradrenaline in the presence of dopamine.

EFFECTS OF CATECHOLAMINES ON RETINAL FUNCTION

Light induces variations in the dopamine content of the retina have been described, but the results are contradictory. In one of the two studies, no statistical evaluation of the change is given (Drujan, Diãz Borges and Alvarez, 1965), and in the other, the significance is only at the five percent level (Nichols, Jacobowitz and Hottenstein, 1967). Adrenaline depletion has been reported in toad retinas exposed to light (Drujan and Diãz Borges, 1968). It should be noted that there are technical difficulties in accurately determining the retinal catecholamines. The total amount of amine in a single retina is below the sensitivity of the common assay procedures, and several retinas must therefore be pooled. Weighing errors, losses during the handling of the tissue in the dark and contamination by vitreous and other tissues also tend to be large and variable. This probably accounts for the discrepancies and the relative sparsity of reports on catecholamine assays on the retina. Some recently developed assay procedures are more sensitive, and useful information is presumably to be expected with them.

Systemic administration of reserpine, which depletes catecholamine stores, makes the animals photophobic. It may be assumed that this is the result of the disappearance of an inhibitory mechanism. However, it is not known whether this is a local effect in the retina or an effect of the central nervous system, although the animals also become photophobic after intraocular injections (Ehinger, 1966). Reserpine has not been found to affect the b wave of the electroretinogram (see Graham, 1973), but Gutierrez and Spiguel (1971) have reported a depression of oscillatory potentials which is perhaps related to the function of the amacrines.

Direct electrophysiological studies of the effect of dopamine on retinal neurons are scarce. When dopamine or noradrenaline is applied to cat ganglion cells electrophoretically or by close intra-arterial injection (Straschill and Perwein, 1969 and 1975), light-evoked excitation is depressed and light-evoked inhibition is enhanced, with no difference for on, off, or on-off cells. In the isolated and perfused rabbit retina (Ames and Pollen, 1969), the responses are more complex. Both α-stimulating and β-stimulating adrenergic drugs increase the activity of off cells and decrease the activity of on and on-off cells. The α-blocker phentolamine has reciprocal effects. This difference between off cells, on the one hand, and on and on-off cells, on the other hand, is intriguing. It is, however, difficult to assess since the drug has been applied to the whole retina rather than to individual cells, so that several and complex synaptic circuits may have been affected.

The above results suggest that dopamine has an inhibitory function in the retina, like it has in most other systems in the central nervous system where this has been tested. Clearly, however, there is a need for much more detailed studies on various aspects of the retinal actions of the catecholamines before a detailed evaluation can be given.

DOPAMINE AS A RETINAL TRANSMITTER

From the chemical assays and the histochemical observations discussed above it is clear that there are high concentrations of dopamine in certain well defined retinal cells. The same neurons are also known to release dopamine upon light stimulation and to recapture it (Kramer, 1971; Kramer, Potts and Magnall, 1971). There appear to be no direct measurements available on dopamine synthesizing systems in the retina. However, dopa decarboxylase inhibition with NSD 1015 almost abolishes the enhancement of specific fluorescence in the retina otherwise caused by l-dopa injections (Ehinger, unpublished), supporting that this enzyme is present. The degrading enzyme, monoamine oxidase, is present (Mizuno, 1960; Eränkö, Niemi and Merenmies, 1961; Mustakallio, 1967). Inhibition of this enzyme results in enhanced fluorescence in the catecholamine containing neurons (Häggendal and Malmfors, 1965). Further, as discussed above, dopamine has clear inhibitory effects on some retinal ganglion cells. Several of the criteria for a neurotransmitter (see chapter 1) are thus fulfilled in the retina for dopamine.

However, some important bits of information are still lacking. We do not know the effect of the neuronal release of endogenous dopamine and therefore cannot compare it with the exogenous application of the substance. This leaves the criterion of identity of action (see chapter 1) still unfulfilled. Also, the responses of individual cells or cell types to dopamine is unknown (except for some ganglion cells), and the precise role of the catecholamine containing neurons can therefore as yet only be guessed at.

5-HYDROXYTRYPTAMINE IN THE RETINA

There are reports of 5-hydroxytryptamine in the retina in the order of a few tenths of micrograms per gram in many species, including rabbits (see: Levine, 1962; Welsh, 1964; Quay, 1965), but Malmfors and Häggendal (1965) were unable to detect any in rabbit retina. In all but one of the studies with the histofluorescence method of Falck and Hillarp, no retinal neurons containing 5-hydroxytryptamine have been reported. The one report is on a special type of cells in chicken retina which appears only during a limited phase of the development (Hauschild and Laties, 1973), and which shows the fluorescence characteristics of an indoleamine such as 5-hydroxytryptamine. No assay has been performed, but some pharmacohistochemical tests were consistent with the presence of an indolamine such as 5-hydroxytryptamine in the neurons. Further, certain indoles have now been found to be preferentially taken up by a set of mammalian retinal amacrine neurons (Ehinger, 1976). These neurons are different from the dopaminergic neurons, but they do not contain enough 5-hydroxytryptamine to make them visible in normal animals. It is not yet known whether 5-hydroxytryptamine or a related indole is the transmitter of these special neurons.

A number of enzymes related to indoleamine metabolism has been reported in the retinas of various animals. Quay (1965) reported varying amounts of hydroxyindole-O-methyltransferase (which forms melatonin from N-acetyl-5-hydroxytryptamine) in fish, amphibians, a turtle (Pseudemys scripta) and leghorn chickens, but little or no enzyme in several other reptiles and birds, and none in rats and monkey retinas. In eyes from growing larvae of the frog Xenopus laevis the enzyme passes a maximum about 8 days after hatching (Barber and Quay, 1969). The enzyme forming 5-hydroxytryptamine by decarboxylating 5-hydroxytryptophan (5-HTPD) falls in the frog at hatching and then rises again (Barber and Quay, 1969). In the mouse, retinal 5-HTPD and hydroxyindole-O-methyltransferase are reported to rise immediately after birth, peaking around the fourth day and then falling to adult levels on about the 7th day (Smith, 1973; Smith and Baker, 1974).

There are few reports on the action of 5-hydroxytryptamine on retinal neurons in vertebrates. Ames and Pollen (1969) find an enhancement of ganglion cell activity of rabbit retinas *in vitro*. In cats, Straschill (1968) reports strong inhibition of ganglion cells by 5-hydroxytryptamine injected in the carotid artery. Microiontophoretic application shows less effect (Straschill and Perwein, 1969 and 1975). These results are not necessarily in conflict, since the application procedures are so different.

The results suggest that there may be a system operating with indoleamines in the mammalian retina. If this is so, the system either has a low transmitter content that makes them difficult to observe, or works with a transmitter that is an indole other than 5-hydroxytryptamine.

It can be added that 5-hydroxytryptamine may be the transmitter of the much studied eccentric cells of the lateral eyes in the horseshoe crab, *Limulus polyphemus* (Adolph, 1966; Adolph and Tuan, 1972; Adolph and Ehinger, 1975).

CONCLUDING REMARKS

Of the biogenic amines, dopamine, noradrenaline, adrenaline and 5-hydroxytryptamine, which are all strong transmitter candidates in the central nervous system, only dopamine can be said to have reached this status in the retina. Generally speaking dopamine seems to have inhibitory activity, presumably in lateral interactions and in feedback loops, although its detailed effects on various parts of the retinal network is not known. Also, one of the main criteria required for its acceptance as a retinal neurotransmitter, that of identify of action, has not yet been satisfied.

There are very marked species differences in the distribution of catecholamine containing neurons, making it imperative to be careful when applying conclusions from one species to another. The recently discovered interplexiform cells may be regarded as good examples: they contain dopamine in most fish and some New World monkeys, but not in Old World monkeys or the common laboratory mammals, where they nevertheless seem to occur. Their transmitter in these cases is unknown.

The dopamine containing interplexiform neurons are interesting in several further ways. They represent a previously unknown pathway in the retina, they occur among others in cold-blooded animals whose tissues are comparatively easy to keep alive *in vitro* and they synapse on the horizontal cells whose electrical signals are comparatively easily monitored.

The variability between species may in some cases be a complication, but it is also of positive interest to the experimenter: by carefully comparing differences in function with differences in morphology, it should be possible to support conclusions about the relations between function and morphology of neurons. However, before this can be done much more knowledge than is presently available has to be collected.

Noradrenaline, adrenaline and 5-hydroxytryptamine cannot at present be regarded as good retinal neurotransmitter candidates, but neither can they be excluded as such, nor are they uninteresting. For both noradrenaline and indoleamines there is sufficient evidence to warrant further investigations as to their possible role in the retina.

ACKNOWLEDGEMENT

This work was supported by the Swedish Medical Research Council, project 04X-2321.

REFERENCES

Adolph A.R. (1966) Excitation and inhibition of electrical activity in the Limulus eye by neuropharmacological agents. In "Functional Organization of the Compound Eye." (C.G. Bernhard, ed.) Pergamon Press, Elmsford, p. 465

Adolph A.R., and Tuan F.J. (1972) Serotonin and inhibition in Limulus lateral eye. J. Gen. Physiol. 60, 679

Adolph A.R., and Ehinger B. (1975) Indoleamines and the eccentric cells of the Limulus lateral eye. Cell and Tissue Research. In press.

Ames A., and Pollen D.A. (1969) Neurotransmission in Central Nervous Tissue: A Study of Isolated Rabbit Retina. J. Neurophysiol. 32, 424

Barker P.C., and Quay W.B. (1969) 5-hydroxytryptamine metabolism in early embryogenesis, and the development of brain and retinal tissues. Brain Research 12, 273

Björklund A., Ehinger B., and Falck B. (1968) A method for differentiating dopamine from noradrenaline in tissue sections by microspectrofluorometry. J. Histochem. Cytochem. 16, 263

Björklund A., Ehinger B. and Falck B. (1972) Analysis of fluorescence excitation peak ratios for the cellular identification of noradrenaline, dopamine, or their mixtures. J. Histochem. Cytochem. 20, 56

Björklund A., Falck B. and Owman Ch. (1972) Fluorescence microscopic and microspectrofluorometric techniques for the cellular localization and characterization of biogenic amines. In "Methods of Investigative and Diagnostic Endocrinology" (J.E. Rall and I. Kopin, eds), North Holland Publ. Corp., The Hague, p. 318

Björklund A. and Falck B. (1973) Cytofluorometry of biogenic monoamines in the Falck-Hillarp method. Structural identification by spectral analysis. In "Fluorescence Techniques in Cell Biology" (A.A. Thaer and M. Sernetz, eds), Springer-Verlag, Berlin-Heidelberg-New York, p. 171

Björklund A., Falck B., Lindvall O. and Svensson L-Å. (1973) New aspects of reaction mechanisms in the formaldehyde histofluorescence method for monoamines. J. Histochem. Cytochem. 21, 17

Boycott B.B., Dowling J.E., Fisher S.K., Kolb H. and Laties A.M. (1975) Interplexiform cells of the mammalian retina and their comparison with catecholamine-containing retinal cells. To be published.

Carlsson A., Dahlström A., Fuxe K. and Hillarp N-Å. (1965) Failure of reserpine to deplete noradrenaline neurons of α-methylnoradrenaline formed from α-methyl DOPA. Acta Pharmacol. Toxicol. 22, 270

Carlsson A., Fuxe K., Hamberger B. and Lindqvist M. (1966) Biochemical and histochemical studies on the effects of imipramine-like drugs and (+)-amphetamine on central and peripheral catecholamine neurons. Acta Physiol. Scand. 67, 481

Carlsson A., Lindqvist M., Fuxe K. and Hökfelt T. (1966) Histochemical and biochemical effects of diethyldithiocarbamate on tissue catecholamines. J. Pharm. Pharmacol. 18, 60

Corrodi H. and Jonsson G. (1967) The formaldehyde fluorescence method for the histochemical demonstration of biogenic monoamines. A review on the methodology. J. Histochem. Cytochem. 15, 65

Curtis D.R. and Johnston G.A.R. (1974) Amino acid transmitters in the mammalian central nervous system. Reviews of Physiology 69, 97

Dowling J.E. (1968) Synaptic organization of the frog retina: an electron microscopic analysis comparing the retinas of frogs and primates. Proc. Roy. Soc. B. 170, 205

Dowling J.E. and Ehinger B. (1975) Synaptic organization of the amine-containing interplexiform cells of the goldfish and Cebus monkey retinas. Science 188, 270

Drujan B.D., Diãz Borges J.M. and Alvarez N. (1965) Relationship between the contents of adrenaline, noradrenaline and dopamine in the retina and its adaptional state. Life Sciences 4, 473

Drujan B.D. and Diãz Borges J.M. (1968) Adrenaline depletion induced by light in the dark-adapted retina. Experientia 24, 674

Ehinger B. (1966) Adrenergic nerves to the eye and to related structures in man and in the cynomolgus monkey. Invest. Ophthalm. 5, 42

Ehinger B. (1967) Adrenergic nerves in the avian eye and ciliary ganglion. Z. Zellforsch. 82, 577

Ehinger B. and Falck B. (1969) Morphological and pharmacohistochemical characteristics of adrenergic retinal neurons and some mammals. Albrecht v. Graefes Arch. klin. exp. Ophthal. 178, 295

Ehinger B. and Falck B. (1969) Adrenergic retinal neurons of some New World monkeys. Z. Zellforsch. 100, 364

Ehinger B., Falck B. and Laties A.M. (1969) Adrenergic neurons in teleost retina. Z. Zellforsch. 97, 285

Ehinger B. (1973) Ocular adrenergic neurons of the flying fox, Pteropus giganteus Brünn (Megachiroptera). Z. Zellforsch. 139, 171

Ehinger B. (1976) Indoleamine accumulating retinal neurons in rabbit and goldfish. To be published.

Eränkö O., Niemi M., and Merenmies E. (1961) Histochemical observations on esterases and oxidative enzymes of the retina. In "The structure of the Eye." (G.K. Smelser, ed.), Acad. Press. New York, p. 159

Eränkö O. (1967) The practical histochemical demonstration of catecholamines by formaldehyde induced fluorescence. J. Royal Microscop. Soc. 87, 259

Falck B. (1962) Observations on the possibilities of the cellular localization of monoamines by a fluorescence method. Acta physiol. Scand. 56, 1

Falck B., Hillarp N., Thieme G., and Torp A. (1962) Fluorescence of catecholamines and related compounds condensed with formaldehyde. J. Histochem. Cytochem. 10, 348

Falck B., Häggendal J., and Owman Ch. (1963) The localization of adrenaline in adrenergic nerves in the frog. Quart. J. Exp. Physiol. XLVIII, 253

Falck B., and Owman Ch. (1965) A detailed methodological description of the fluorescence method for the cellular demonstration of biogenic monoamines. Acta Univ. Lund Sectio II, No. 7, p. 1

Graham L.T. (1973) Comparative aspects of neurotransmitters in the retina. In "The Eye.", vol. 6 (Davson H. and Graham L.T., eds.) Acad. Press, New York, p. 283

Gutierrez C.O., and Spiguel R.D. (1973) Oscillatory potentials of the cat retina: Effects of adrenergic drugs. Life Sciences, 13, 991

Häggendal J., and Malmfors T. (1963) Evidence of dopamine-containing neurons in the retina of the rabbit. Acta physiol. Scand. 59, 295

Häggendal J., and Malmfors T. (1965) Identification and cellular localization in the retina and the chorioid of the rabbit. Acta physiol. Scand. 64, 58

Hauschild D., and Laties A.M. (1973) An indoleamine-containing cell in chick retina. Invest. Ophthal. 12, 537

Hökfelt T. (1967) On the ultrastructural localization of noradrenaline in the central nervous system of the rat. Z. Zellforsch. Mikroskop. Anat. 79, 110

Hökfelt T. (1968) In vitro studies on central and peripheral monoamine neurons at the ultrastructural level. Z. Zellforsch. Mikroskop. Anat. 91, 1

Hökfelt T., and Jonsson G. (1968) Studies on reaction and binding of monoamines after fixation and processing for electron microscopy with special reference to fixation with potassium permanganate. Histochemie 16, 45

Kramer S.G. (1971) Dopamine: A retinal neurotransmitter. I. Retinal uptake, storage, and light-stimulated release of H^3-dopamine in vivo. Invest. Ophthal. 10:6, 438

Kramer S.G., Potts A.M., and Magnall Y. (1971) Dopamine: A retinal neurotransmitter. II. Autoradiographic localization of H^3-dopamine in the retina. Invest. Ophthal. 10, 617

Krnjevič K. (1974) Chemical nature of synaptic transmission in vertebrates. Physiol. Rev. 54, 418

Laties A., and Jacobowitz D. (1966) A comparative study of the autonomic innervation of the eye in monkey, cat and rabbit. Anat. Rec. 156, 383

Levene R.Z. (1962) Mast cells and amines in normal ocular tissues. Invest. Ophthal. 1, 531

Malmfors T. (1963) Evidence of adrenergic neurons with synaptic terminals in the retina of rats demonstrated with fluorescence and electron microscopy. Acta physiol. Scand. 58, 99

Mizuno K. (1960) Studies on retinitis pigmentosa. I. Monoamine oxidase and sulfase conjugation in the experimental degeneration of the retina. Eye, Ear, Nose and Throat. 39 493

Mustakallio A. (1967) Monoamine oxidase activity in the various structures of the mammalian eye. Histochemical staining and quantitative chemical study. Acta Ophthal. 93, 1

Nichols S., Jacobowitz D., and Hottenstein M. (1967) The influence of light and dark on the catecholamine content of the retina and choroid. Invest. Ophthal. 6, 642

Pellegrino de Iraldi A., and Etcheverry G.J. (1967) Granulated vesicles in retinal synapses and neurons. Z. Zellforsch. Mikroskop. Anat. 81, 283

Quay W.B. (1965) Retinal and pineal hydroxyindole - o - methyl transferase activity in vertebrates. Life Sci. 4, 983

Quay W.B. (1965) Indole derivatives of pineal and related neural and retinal tissues. Pharmacol. Rev. 17, 321

Sano Y., Yoshikawa H., and Konishi M. (1968) Fluorescence microscopic observations on the dog retina. Arch. Histol. Jap. 30, 75

Scheie E., and Laties A.M. (1971) Catecholamine-containing cells in the retinas of Gekko Gecko and Rana Pipiens. Herpetologica. 27, 77

Smith M.D. (1973) 5-hydroxytryptamine decarboxylase (5-HTPD) and monoamine oxidase (MAO) in the maturing mouse eye. Comp. Gen. Pharmacol. 4, 175

Smith M.D., and Baker P.C. (1974) The maturation of melantonin synthesis in the lateral eyes of the mouse. Comp. Gen. Pharmacol. 5, 275

Stell W.K. (1972) The morphological organization of the vertebrate retina. In "Handbook of Sensory Physiology" (M.G.F. Fuortes, ed.), vol. VII/2, Springer-Verlag, Berlin, p. 111

Straschill M. (1968) Actions of drugs on single neurons in the cat's retina. Vision Res. 8, 35

Straschill M., and Perwein J. (1969) The inhibition of retinal ganglion cells by catecholamines and γ-aminobutyric acid. Pflügers Arch. Europ. J. Physiol. 312, 45

Straschill M., and Perwein J. (1975) Effects of biogenic amines and amino acids on the cat's retinal ganglion cells. In: Proceedings of the Golgi Centennial Symposium (ed: M. Santini). Raven Press, 583

Welsh J.H. (1964) The quantitative distribution of 5-hydroxytryptamine in the nervous system, eyes and other organs of some vertebrates. In: Comp. Neurochem. Proc. of the 5th Internat. Neurochem. Symp., Pergamon Press. 25, 355

Werman R. (1972) Amino acids as central neurotransmitters. Res. Publ. Assoc. Res. Nerv. Ment. Dis. 50, 147

CHAPTER 8

DOPAMINE IN RETINAL NEUROTRANSMISSION

Steven G. Kramer, M.D., Ph.D.
University of California, San Francisco
Department of Ophthalmology
and
Veterans Administration Hospital, San Francisco
Ophthalmology Service

INTRODUCTION

Over a decade ago, Haggendal and Malmfors (1965) noted that laboratory animals treated with reserpine showed photophobia. It was reasoned that the drug might have induced depletion of a biogenic amine in the retina (Carlsson, 1966), and that if such an amine were acting as an inhibitory chemical neurotransmitter, its depletion would account for the photophobia. Blockade of an aminergic inhibitory transmitter system could be expected to increase retinal sensitivity.

Haggendal and Malmfors (1965) studied the retina with the use of the histochemical fluorescent technique of Falck and Owman (1965), which provides accurate anatomical localization of intraneuronal catecholamines. They identified a layer of catecholamine-containing fibers and cell bodies at the junction of the retinal inner nuclear and inner plexiform layers in several species. By the chemical analysis (Haggendal, 1967) of pooled rabbit retinas (Haggendal and Malmfors, 1965), they identified the catecholamine present as dopamine. Nichols and colleagues (Nichols et al., 1967) confirmed that the retinal catecholamine was dopamine in rabbits, guinea pigs, and rats; norepinephrine, on the other hand, was virtually absent.

Elegant histochemical studies have characterized this system of retinal dopamine-containing neurons (Ehinger, 1966; Laties and Jacobowitz, 1966 a and b; Sano, Yoshikawa and Konishi, 1968; Ehinger, Falck and Laties, 1969; Ehinger and Falck, 1969). They are similar in morphology to amacrine cells, although numerically they comprise only about ten per cent of these cells (Ehinger, 1966). Recently, Ehinger and Falck (1969) have proposed the term "adrenergic junctional cells" to identify those amacrine-like cells at the junction of the inner nuclear and inner plexiform layers which contain catecholamines.

The modifier "adrenergic" is used descriptively in this case, but in theory it should not be applied unless the cells in question have been shown to utilize "noradrenalin" (norepinephrine) as their neurotransmitter. The results reported in the present paper suggest that the "junctional cells" actually release dopamine as their neurotransmitter, that the dopamine acts as an inhibitory transmitter, and that the cells are in fact "dopaminergic junctional cells" with inhibitory function. They are cells which are completely independent of the ocular sympathetics, which innervate the uveal tract and blood vessels, and they are probably functionally distinct from other amacrine cells.

Classically, neuropharmacologists have accepted a set of fairly rigid criteria which must be established in order to identify any substance as a neurotransmitter (Curtis, 1961; McLennan, 1963). This group of "Koch's postulates" of chemical transmission is given in Table 8.1 in summarized form.

Table 8.1. Criteria Required to Identify any Substance, X, as a Neurotransmitter of a Specific Neuron

Criterion
1. Presence of X in the neuron
2. Presence of mechanisms for synthesis and degradation of X in the neuron
3. Release of X when the neuron is stimulated
4. Discharge (or inhibition) of the postsynaptic neuron by direct application of X
5. Pharmacologic "blockers" of X at other sites should block the physiologic action of the neuron

With respect to retinal dopamine, this chapter will present evidence in support of criteria 2, 3 and 5, and will review available evidence in support of criteria 1 and 4.

In support of criterion 2, the first part of the present chapter describes <u>carotid infusion</u> of radioactive dopamine followed by radiochemical analysis of extracts of the retinal tissue. In support of criterion 3, the second and third parts of the chapter describe <u>preretinal perfusion</u> with radioactive dopamine, a technique which demonstrates uptake and release of dopamine from the living retina. Storage and localization are confirmed by autoradiography.

CAROTID INFUSION STUDIES

Materials

Radiochemicals used in these studies included chromatographically pure tritiated dopamine (H3-DA), tritiated norepinephrine (H3-NE), and tritiated normetanephrine (H3-NM), all obtained from the New England Nuclear Corporation, Boston, Mass. Nonradioactive chemicals included dopamine (DA), norepinephrine (NE), normetanephrine (NM), dihydroxyphenylacetic acid (DPA) and homovanillic acid (HVA), obtained from the Nutritional Biochemicals Corporation, Cleveland, Ohio.

Major equipment used in the experiments included a Packard model 3375 Tri-Carb Liquid Scintillation Spectrometer, a Packard model 7201 Radiochromatogram scanner, a Packard model 34 Fraction Collector, a Zeiss model II operating microscope, two Sigmamotor model AL-2E infusion pumps, a Harvard model 661 small animal respirator, a Grass model S4 stimulator coupled to a General Radio Strobolume stroboscope, a clinical electroretinography recording system described previously (Krill, Potts and Johanson, 1971), a Virtis model 10-146MR-BA Freeze-Mobile lyophilizer, and a Servall refrigerated centrifuge.

Methods

General experimental design. The plan was essentially similar to that of experiments described previously (Kramer and Potts, 1969 a and b). In brief, tritiated catecholamines (either H3-DA or H3-NE) were infused for 30 minutes into the right carotid arteries of six adult female cats weighing 2 to 3 kilograms. The animals were killed, and both eyes were removed. The eyes were dissected, the iris, ciliary body, choroid, and retina were weighed, and the total radioactivity in each of these tissues was measured. Similar experiments were done in six animals at varying intervals after complete right superior cervical ganglionectomy. Measurements were made in one animal at one day, one at six days, one at twelve days, and in three at twenty days after ganglionectomy. In one additional animal subjected to H3-DA infusion, the retina was frozen, and an acidified acetone extraction of the frozen tissue was done; quantitative paper radiochromatography of this tissue was then performed.

Catecholamine infusion technique, radioactivity analysis, and ganglionectomy technique. Each of these methods has been described in detail in previous papers (Kramer and Potts, 1969 a and b).

Acidified acetone extraction. The method was a modification of the extraction procedure of Fleming and associates (Fleming et al., 1965), suggested in part by Halushka and Hoffman (1968). The technique can be described as follows:

Redistilled acetone was used to make acidified acetone immediately before use by shaking 100 ml of the acetone with an excess of sodium metabisulfite as an antioxidant. The suspension was filtered, and concentrated HCl (1 ml) was added to the filtrate.

After completion of carotid infusion of H3-DA and dissection of the eye, the retina was washed in ice-cold saline, placed on an aluminium foil spatula, and frozen in liquid nitrogen. The frozen retina was crushed under liquid nitrogen, and each succeeding step was done at 4° C. under a nitrogen atmosphere. The particles of frozen tissue were homogenized in a motor-driven microhomogenizer containing ice-cold acetone (2 ml) which contained nonradioactive carrier dopamine, norepinephrine, dihydroxyphenylacetic acid, and homovanillic acid (100 μg each). The homogenizer was washed twice with acidified acetone (0.5 ml), and the washings were added to the original homogenate.

The mixture was transferred to a plastic centrifuge tube which was flushed with nitrogen and capped. The homogenate was centrifuged for 10 minutes at 20,000 r.p.m. in the refrigerated centrifuge, and the supernatant was brought to a final volume of 4 ml by the addition of further acidified acetone. This was evaporated to near dryness in a flash evaporator. Ice-cold n-butanol (2 ml) saturated with 0.01 N HCl containing 0.1 per cent ethylenediamine tetraacetic acid (EDTA) was added, and the combination was mixed under nitrogen for three minutes. N-Heptane (4 ml) and 0.01 N HCl (1 ml) containing 0.01 per cent EDTA was added, followed by further mixing under nitrogen for three minutes. The n-butanolheptane layer was separated by centrifugation at 5,000 r.p.m. for five minutes in a capped tube which had been flushed with nitrogen, and this layer was aspirated off. The remaining HCl layer was then freeze-dried in the Virtis lyophilizer; the frozen sample was stored under nitrogen and later reconstituted with a 5:1 mixture of acetone (0.25 ml) and 0.01 N HCl. This mixture (50 μl) was spotted for chromatography.

In preliminary experiments, recovery of H3-DA, H3-NE, and H3-NM, added to the original tissue specimens, varied between 85 and 95 per cent. Radiochemical purity did not vary significantly from that of the original compounds.

Radiochromatography. Strips of Whatman No. 1 filter paper were prepared by saturation (Goldbaum and Kazyak, 1956) with 0.067 M phosphate buffer mixed in 1 per cent sodium metabisulfite instead of water with the final pH adjusted to 6.8 (Halushka, 1967). The extract (50 μl) was spotted under nitrogen at the origin of each strip approximately 3 μl at a time. A 50 μl standard mixture containing dopamine, norepinephrine, normetanephrine, dihydroxyphenylacetic acid, and homovanillic acid (50μg each), as well as H3-DA, H3-NE, and H3-NM (0.1 μc), was spotted on a different chromatogram strip, but run at the same time.

The chromatographic solvent was butanol: acetic acid:water (4:1:1) (Whitby, Axelrod and Weil-Malherbe, 1961), and large strips of filter paper saturated with this mixture were used to line the chromatograph tank. The tank was flushed with nitrogen through a long glass tube, and the spotted strips were allowed to equilibrate with the nitrogen-solvent atmosphere for three hours. Solvent was then added to the chromatograph trough for descending chromatography lasting eight to ten hours.

The strips were air dried and sprayed with 0.44 per cent potassium ferricyanide in 0.1 M phosphate buffer with a pH of 7.6 to develop the spots (Bertler, Carlsson and Rosengren, 1958). Dopamine, norepinephrine, and dihydroxyphenylacetic acid gave light lavender spots on a yellow background, and normetanephrine and homovanillic acid gave white spots on a yellow background. Both colors were enhanced for purposes of detection by viewing them in ultraviolet light.

After measurements to determine R_f values were made, the chromatogram strips were scanned on the Packard radiochromatogram scanner in order to measure the radioactivity associated with each spot. The resultant curves were integrated with an Ott planimeter.

Data processing and display of data. A computer program to make calculations of all data on this and other similar radioactivity studies was written. The results were automatically displayed as bar graphs or curves on a cathode-ray oscilloscope connected to the computer, and 35 mm slides of the oscilloscope face were made. Most of the figures in this chapter, therefore, are reproductions of computer-generated oscilloscope displays. Centering, scaling, plotting, and numerial and alphabetic labeling were all done automatically and, for practical purposes, instantaneously.

Results

Fig. 8.1 illustrates the total retention of radioactivity in the retinas of six animals (expressed in terms of millimicromoles of infused substance per gram of retina) following carotid infusion of H3-DA or H3-NE. The amount of retention is exceedingly small but clearly different on the side of infusion from that on the opposite side.

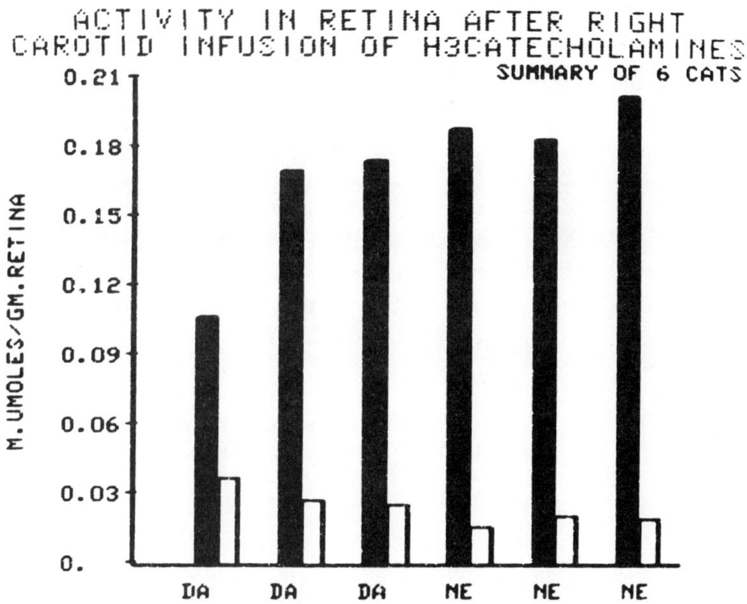

Fig. 8.1. Closed bars--infused side; open bars--non-infused side.

As shown in Fig. 8.2, when the experiment was repeated in six animals at intervals after superior cervical ganglionectomy, there was no difference in retention from that before ganglionectomy. This is in contradistinction to sympathetically innervated tissues of the anterior segment (Kramer and Potts, 1969 a and b).

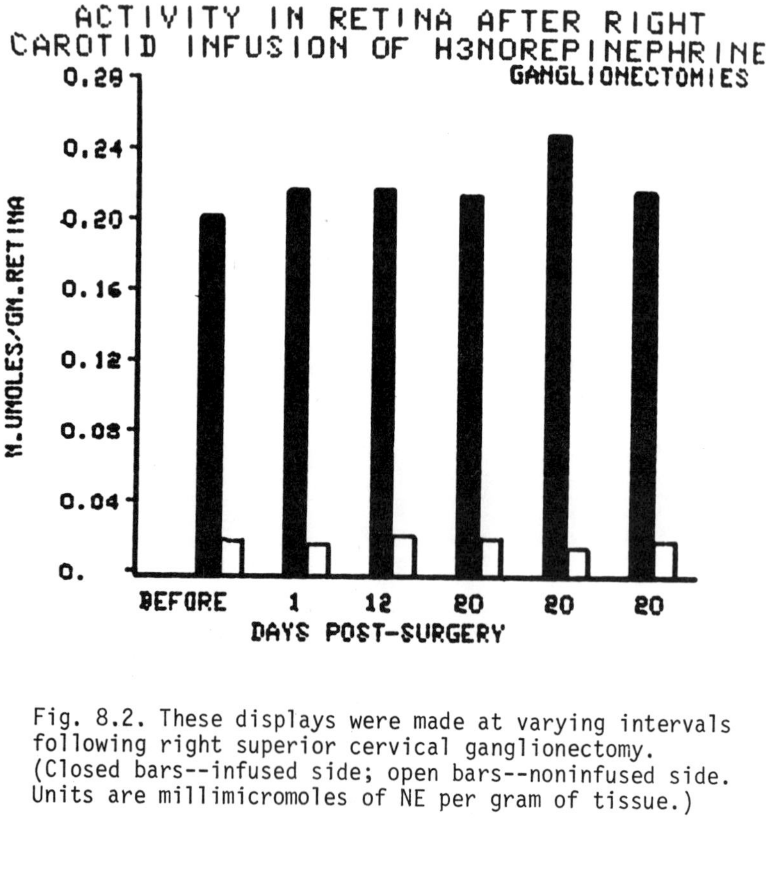

Fig. 8.2. These displays were made at varying intervals following right superior cervical ganglionectomy. (Closed bars--infused side; open bars--noninfused side. Units are millimicromoles of NE per gram of tissue.)

Radiochromatography on the acidified-acetone extract of the retina is illustrated in Fig. 8.3. Activity migrated on the chromatogram strip in association with authentic dopamine (32 per cent of total), dihydroxyphenylacetic acid (18 per cent), norepinephrine (15 per cent), and homovanillic acid (15 per cent). Virtually no activity was associated with normetanephrine.

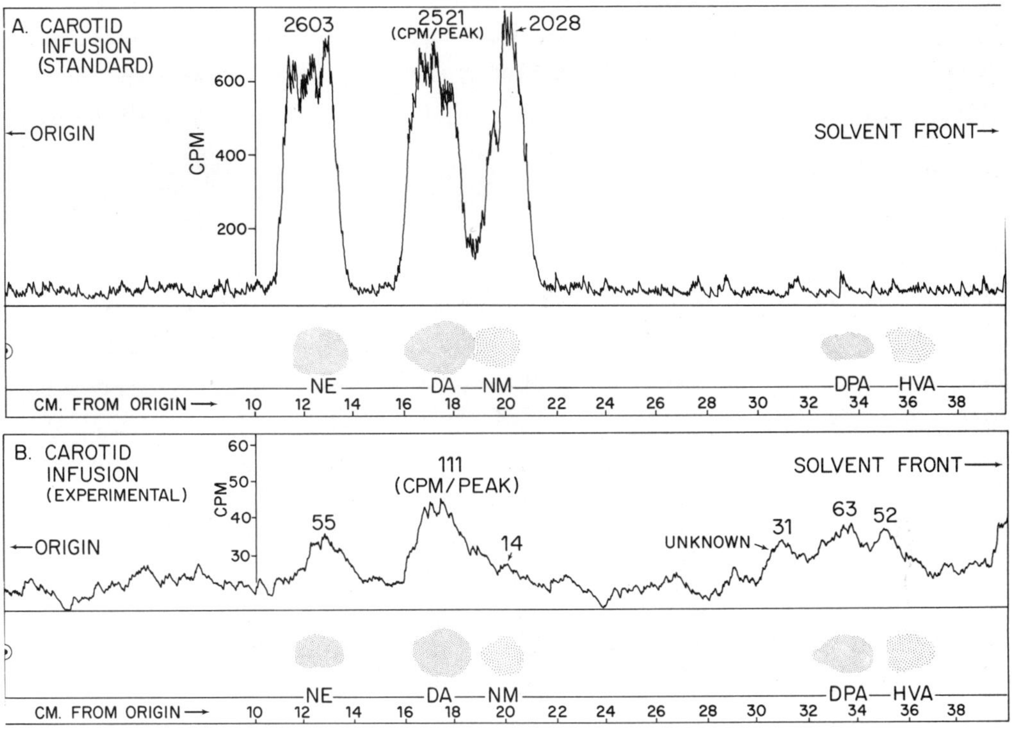

Fig. 8.3. Radiochromatography of acidified acetone retinal extract following right carotid infusion of H3-DA. (A) Tracing of standard chromatogram; (B) tracing of experimental chromatogram of extract run simultaneously with standard. (SCAN) Recorder output from radiochromatogram scanner; (STRIP) chromatogram strip; spots are tracings of actual spots on chromatogram strips. (CPM) Counts per minute; (NE) norepinephrine; (DA) dopamine; (NM) normetanephrine; (DPA) dihydroxyphenylacetic acid; and (HVA) homovanillic acid. Number above peak indicates area under peak or CPM per peak.

PRE-RETINAL PERFUSION STUDIES

Materials

See under "Carotid infusion studies", p. 168.

Methods

General experimental design. In order to demonstrate and measure uptake and light stimulated release of H3-DA from retinal neurons in vivo, an experimental preparation in the cat eye, called preretinal perfusion, was developed (Fig. 8.4). The exposed retinal surface was perfused with an isotonic solution containing H3-DA, and the radioactivity of precise aliquots of the perfusate was monitored as a function of time during perfusion. A drop in radioactivity level of the effluent perfusate was considered indicative of uptake of H3-DA from the perfusate. Subsequent continuation of perfusion with the same concentration of nonradioactive dopamine allowed measurement of a steady-state, low, background level of radioactivity in the effluent perfusate. During this continued perfusion with nonradioactive dopamine, the retina was stimulated by an intermittent flashing stimulus with the use of the Strobolume. Any resultant increase in radioactivity above background in the effluent perfusate was considered indicative of release of H3-DA induced by the light stimulus.

Three adult cats weighing 2 to 3 kilograms were used in each of five experimental groups based on the rate of the flashing stimulus and the state of retinal light-dark adaptation (Table 8.2). In one animal of each experimental

Table 8.2. Grouping of Animals for Preretinal Perfusion

Group	No. of cats	Conditions
I	3	Dark -adapted, stimulus rate = 1 flash/2 sec.
II	3	Dark -adapted, stimulus rate = 1 flash/sec.
III	3	Dark -adapted, stimulus rate = 2 flashes/sec.
IV	3	Light-adapted, stimulus rate = 1 flash/2 sec.
V	3	Light-adapted, stimulus rate = 2 flashes/sec.

group, bilateral optic nerve section was performed before initiating preretinal perfusion. Two additional cats were used, one light-adapted and one dark-adapted, in which preretinal perfusion was carried out, but no flashing stimulus was given.

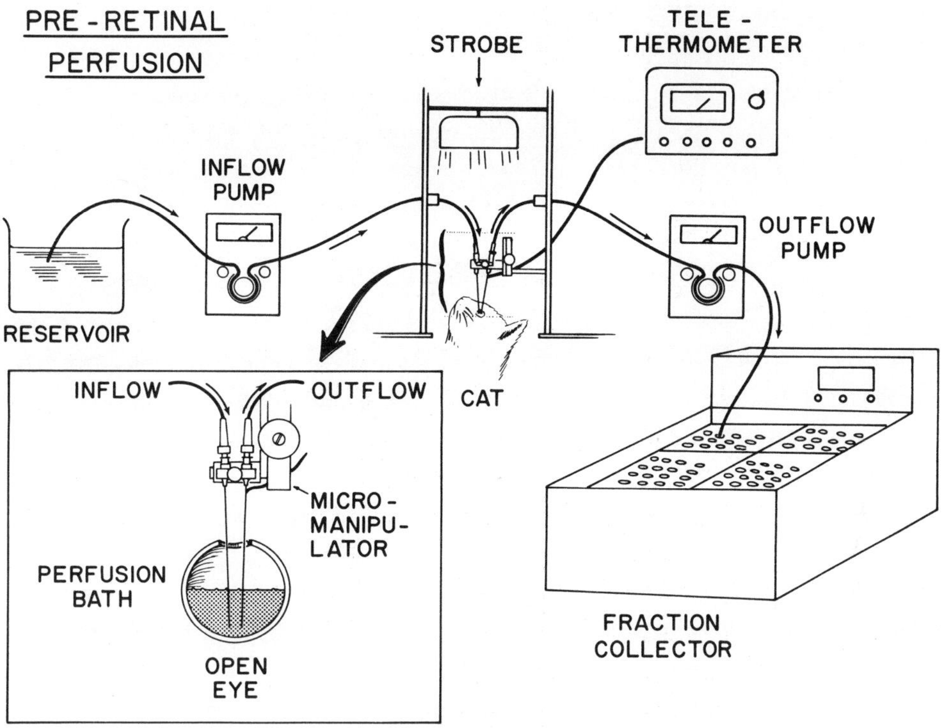

Fig. 8.4. Schematic diagram of preretinal perfusion preparation.

Although small perfusate aliquots were used to monitor radioactivity as a function of time during perfusion, most of the perfusate obtained during light stimulation was saved and frozen under conditions designed to prevent oxidative change of the perfusate constituents. These frozen perfusate samples were pooled at the conclusion of all the experiments and were analyzed by radiochromatography in order to identify the radioactive components.

Preparation of animals and surgical techniques. Each animal was anesthetized with sodium pentobarbital (30 mg per kilogram of body weight) administered intraperitoneally. A simple tracheotomy was performed, and a Y-tube was tied into the trachea and connected to a Harvard respirator. The right femoral vein was exposed and cannulated with a PE No. 160 polyethylene catheter. The head was fixed with a clamp so that the left eye was directed upward with its equatorial plane parallel with the ceiling. A large lateral canthotomy was performed, and the lids were secured with 4-0 black silk sutures. The nictitating membrane was removed, and a 360° conjunctival peritomy at the limbus was done. The anterior chamber was entered by an ab externo scratch incision, and the entire cornea was removed with corneoscleral scissors.

The iris was dilated mechanically by rupturing the sphincter with the use of iris retractors. The anterior lens capsule was cut with a scalpel blade and stripped away using capsule forceps and scissors. The lens nucleus and cortex were removed with a lens loop, thereby exposing the posterior lens capsule. The posterior capsule and anterior hyaloid were grasped gently with capsule forceps and cut with iris scissors.

Total removal of the vitreous was accomplished in three stages: (1) The major portion of the solid vitreous was removed piecemeal by very gentle traction with Weck surgical cellulose sponges, followed by cutting with iris scissors as described by Kasner (1968). (2) The remaining vitreous was then disorganized by repeated scissors snips into the gel without any attempt at removal. (3) Following this disorganization, virtually all remaining vitreous could be removed with the use of gentle suction with a glass cannula (Pasteur pipette). Retinal trauma was minimized by virtue of the high magnification available with the operating microscope. At any stage of the procedure, overly vigorous traction on the vitreous was found to produce immediate retinal detachment. Only preparations without detachment or retinal hemorrhage and with intact circulation were used for perfusion.

Intracranial bilateral optic nerve section was done before perfusion in one animal of each experimental group. A wide frontal craniotomy was done, the frontal lobes were retracted, and both optic nerves were severed with a Bovie electrocautery blade. Subsequently, preretinal perfusion was carried out as in all other animals.

Perfusion apparatus. As indicated in Fig. 8.4, the apparatus included a reservoir, an inflow tubing connected to a Sigmamotor stripping pump with a continuously variable speed control, a pair of 22 guage inflow and outflow needles attached to a micromanipulator, an outflow tubing connected to an

Table 8.3. Phases of Preretinal Perfusion*

Phase	Time (min.)	Perfusate
Uptake	0-20	H3-DA
Washout	21-30	Nonradioactive dopamine in same molar concentration
Release[x]	31-60	Nonradioactive dopamine in same molar concentration

*Rate of perfusion = 1 ml per minute
[x]Light stimulation given in release phase. See Groups I to V, Table 8.2.

identical Sigmamotor pump, and a fraction collector to isolate aliquots of the perfusate. During perfusion, fluid was pumped from the reservoir through the inflow needle into the open eye, over the exposed retinal surface, and out of the eye via the outflow needle to the fraction collector. A small flexible thermistor was attached to the tip of the outflow needle to allow continuous monitoring of the temperature of the intraocular perfusate on a Yellow Springs Telethermometer.

A flashing stimulus was provided by a General Radio Corporation Strobolume set at low intensity and triggered externally by a Grass stimulator. The center of the face of the lamp housing was positioned eight inches from the exposed retina. During perfusion, no change in the temperature of the perfusate in the eye was induced by the flashing stimulus.

Phases of perfusion and state of adaptation. The three phases of perfusion are summarized in Table 8.3. The rate of perfusion throughout was kept constant at 1 ml per minute. During the first or "uptake" phase, the perfusion fluid consisted of isotonic saline (20 ml) containing H3-DA (40 μc), with a specific activity of 3,600 μc per millimole, and sodium heparin (100 USP units). At the end of this phase, fluid in the entire system was exchanged for isotonic saline containing nonradioactive dopamine and heparin in the same molar concentrations as existed in the original fluid. The fluid within the eye itself was exchanged three times with the use of a Pasteur pipette. Perfusion was then continued for an additional 10 minutes during the second or "washout phase". During the third or "release phase", perfusion was continued for 30 minutes without changing the perfusion fluid, but a flashing stimulus was added at a rate of 1 flash per 2 seconds, 1 flash per second, or 2 flashes per second, depending on the experiment (Table 8.2).

Light-adapted animals were kept in the ordinary room illumination of the laboratory throughout the experiment. Dark-adapted animals were put in total darkness 15 minutes before initiating perfusion and were kept in the dark until conclusion of the experiment. A Kodak Safelight, Wratten No. 2, was used during exchange of the perfusion fluid at the beginning of the "washout phase" and intermittently for checks on the status of the preparation. The laboratory was light tight, instrument lights were masked, and the preparation was covered with a heavy felt canopy during dark adaptation.

Electroretinography. A previously described clinical electroretinography unit (Krill, Potts and Johanson, 1971) was used to record the electroretinogram (ERG) in three animals after vitrectomy but before perfusion and again after completion of perfusion. The recording electrode was a Ag-AgCl wick electrode in contact with the perfusion fluid, and the reference electrode was a needle electrode in the frontalis muscle. The stimulus was provided by the Strobolume discussed above, and the oscilloscope sweep was triggered by the syncopated output of the Grass stimulator with a 20 msec. delay. That the retina remains electrophysiologically intact during the experiments is supported by a normal ERG after vitrectomy, both before and after perfusion (Fig. 8.5).

Collection, storage, and analysis of perfusate samples. The fraction collector was programmed to collect approximately 0.15 and 1 ml of perfusate in alternate tubes (one pair of tubes per minute) by counting microdrops. The 0.15 ml aliquots were used for direct radioactivity measurement, and the 1 ml aliquots were used for radiochromatography.

A micropipette was used to aspirate precisely 0.1 ml from each 0.15 ml aliquot tube, and this was transferred to another tube containing a 4:1 mixture of ethanol and methanol (4 ml). After mixing, this solution (1 ml) was transferred to a scintillation counting vial containing scintillant (15 ml) with the following composition: 0.4 per cent 2,5-diphenyloxazol and 0.01 per cent B-bis(2(phenyloxazolyl)) benzene in toluene (w/v). The radioactivity of the

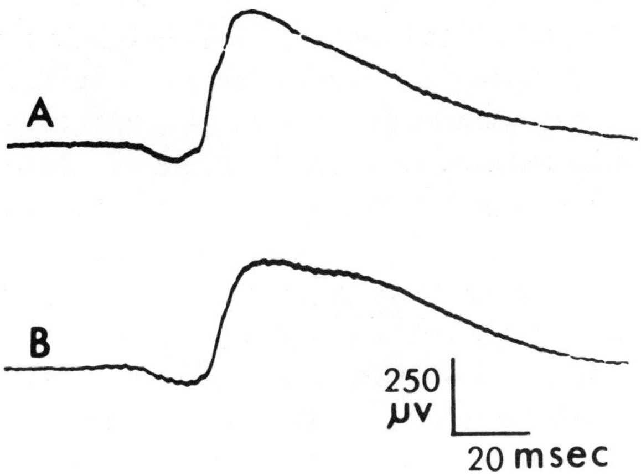

Fig. 8.5. Single electroretinographic response after vitrectomy in preretinal perfusion preparation. (A) Before perfusion; (B) after perfusion.

mixture was measured in the Tri-Carb Liquid Scintillation Spectrometer. Standards with known concentrations of H3-DA were prepared and analyzed by the same technique.

The 1 ml aliquots from the 30 minute "release phase" (Table 8.3) were pooled and brought to a final total volume of 30 ml. To this were added nonradioactive dopamine, norepinephrine, normetanephrine, dihydroxyphenylacetic acid, and homovanillic acid (10 μg each). The 30 ml mixture was freeze-dried in the Virtis lyophilizer, and the frozen powder was stored in a nitrogen atmosphere at -15° C.

After completion of the experimental series, the pooled frozen specimens from the release phases of all 15 experiments were each reconstituted with a 5:1 mixture of acetone and 0.01 N HCl (0.3 ml) and a pooled mixture of all the samples was made. The mixture was evaporated under vacuum, and the residue was reconstitued with acetone-HCl (0.25 ml). The final solution (50 μl) was chromatographed as in Part I.

Autoradiography. Small pieces of sclerachoroid-retina from the fixed eyes were cut and washed in cold phosphate buffer for 15 minutes. The tissues were postfixed in two per cent osmium tetroxide in cold buffer for three hours and were dehydrated and embedded in Epon. One-micron sections were cut, heated, and cooled until they adhered to cleaned, glass slides.

Under Safelight conditions (Wratten No. 2), the slides were dipped in Ilford K-5 nuclear emulsion, dried, and stored in black plastic slide boxes containing 50 to 100 mg of dried silica gel. The emulsion overlying the sections was photographically developed at one-week intervals over a six-week period and at one-month intervals thereafter. In glass slide-racks in total darkness and at 70^{0} C., the slides were sequentially dipped in Kodak D-19 developer for two minutes, distilled water for 20 seconds, and Edwal Quick-fix photographic fixer for 30 seconds. They were washed in three changes of distilled water for a total of five minutes, and the sections were stained through the emulsion for 30 seconds with a mixture of toluidine blue and pyronin B. When the emulsion was too heavily stained, destaining was done with ten per cent ethyl alcohol or two per cent polyvinyl alcohol. Coverslips were applied with Preservaslide mounting medium (Matheson, Coleman, and Bell), and photomicrographs were taken with a Zeiss photomicroscope.

Control slides from animals not subjected to catecholamine perfusion or infusion were prepared and treated identically. Such controls for each tissue accompanied experimental tissues during each step of exposure and development.

Results

Uptake and release. Radioactivity analysis of the perfusate obtained during the "uptake phase" of preretinal perfusion (Table 8.3) is shown in Fig. 8.6,A. The decrease in activity of the perfusate during the first ten minutes suggests extraction of H3-DA from the fluid by the preparation; subsequent return of activity toward the original level during the second ten minutes suggests saturation of the preparation.

The radioactivity level of the perfusate during the "washout phase" (Table 8.3) is shown in Fig. 8.6,B. The progressive drop in activity to a low back-

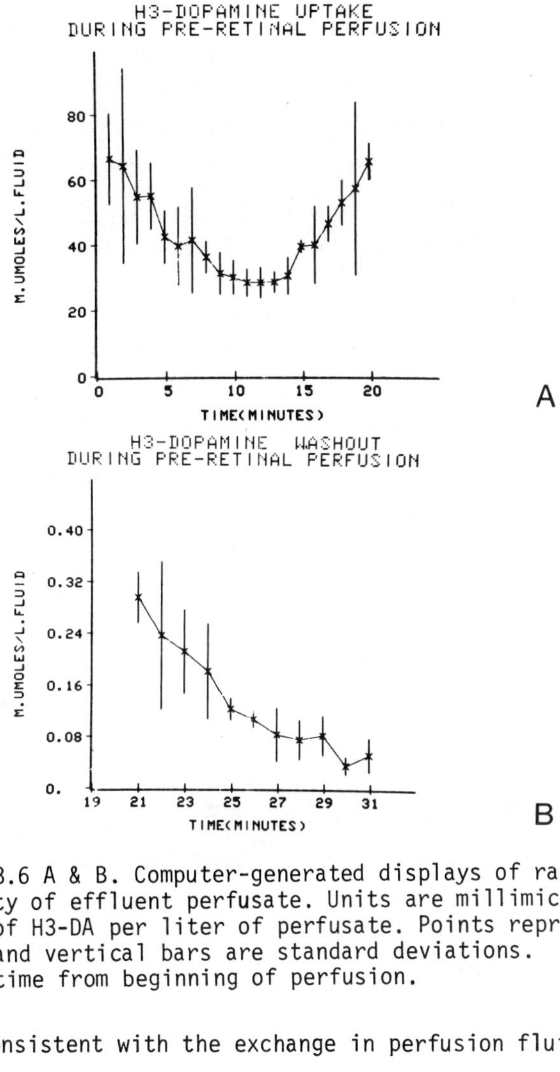

Figs. 8.6 A & B. Computer-generated displays of radioactivity of effluent perfusate. Units are millimicromoles of H3-DA per liter of perfusate. Points represent means and vertical bars are standard deviations. Time: time from beginning of perfusion.

ground level is consistent with the exchange in perfusion fluid to that containing nonradioactive dopamine.

Perfusate radioactivity level during the "release phase" (Table 8.3), or the phase during which retinal light stimulation is given, is shown in Figs. 8.7 and 8.8, which represent data from animals in Groups I to V (Table 8.2). Fig. 8.7 shows the results from animals which were dark-adapted, but in which the flashing stimulus rate was either 1 per 2 seconds, 1 per second, or 2 per second. It is apparent that the flashing stimulus induces an increase in perfusate radioactivity, and the rate of this increase in activity increases with increasing rate of stimulation.

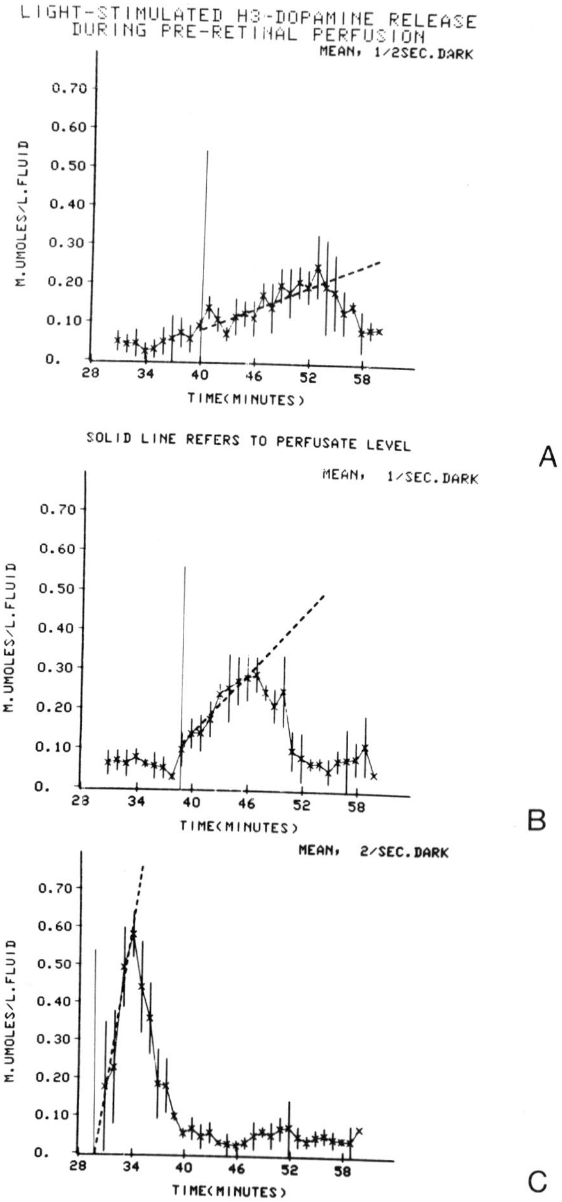

Figs. 8.7 A, B & C. Computer-generated display of radioactivity of effluent perfusate during "release phase" of preretinal perfusion in <u>dark-adapted</u> animals. (A) Group I: stimulus rate--1 flash/2 seconds; (B) Group II: stimulus rate--1 flash/second; (C) Group III: stimulus rate--2 flashes/second. Units are millimicromoles of H3-DA per liter of perfusate. Points represent means of three animals, and vertical bars are standard deviations. Time: time from beginning of perfusion.

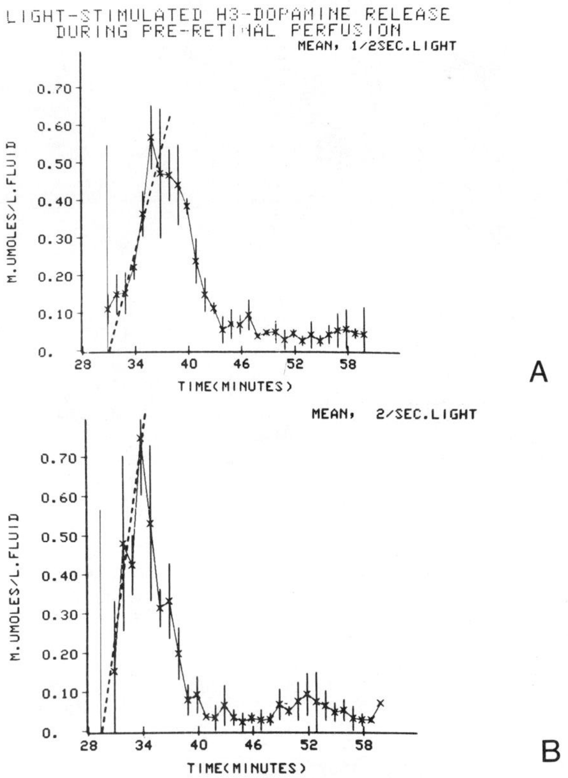

Figs. 8.8 A & B. Computer-generated display of radioactivity of effluent perfusate during "release phase" of preretinal perfusion in light-adapted animals. (A) Group IV: stimulus rate--1 flash/2 seconds; (B) Group V: stimulus rate--2 flashes/second. Units are millimicromoles of H3-DA per liter of perfusate. Points represent means of three animals, and vertical bars are standard deviations. Time: time from beginning of perfusion.

A least-squares straight-line fit of the points during the period of increasing radioactivity was done and is indicated by a heavy dotted line in each figure. The slope of this line gives the rate of release of the perfusate radioactivity and is a function of the rate of release of activity from the preparation into the perfusate. The slope of the line, or the rate of release, increases disproportionately with the increase in stimulus rate.

Fig. 8.8 shows similar data during the "release phase" for experiments done on light-adapted animals from Groups IV and V (Table 8.2), with stimulus rates of 1 per 2 seconds and 2 per second. There is again a marked release of

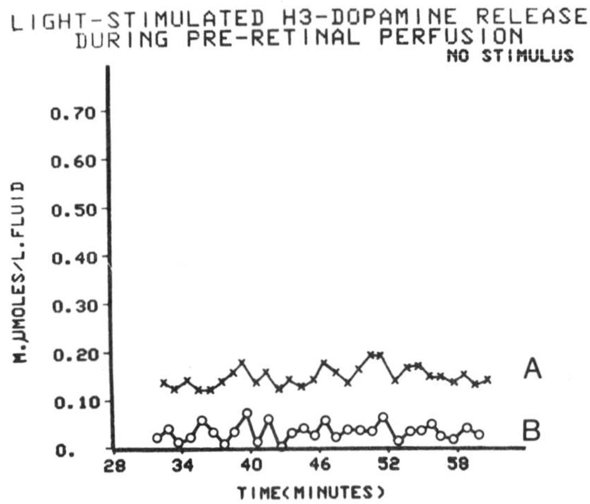

Fig. 8.9. Dopamine release in light-adapted (A) and dark-adapted (B) animals in millimicromoles H3-DA per liter perfusate. Time: time from beginning of perfusion.

activity into the perfusate by the preparation, induced apparently by the flashing stimulus, but the rate of release (slope of the fitted line) is not related clearly to the stimulus frequency. Furthermore, the rate at the slowest frequency is much greater than it was in dark-adapted animals at the same frequency (compare Figs. 8.7, A and 8.8, A).

Fig. 8.9 shows perfusate radioactivity levels from two animals, one dark- and one light-adapted, in which perfusion was continued, but no flashing stimulus was used. While the light-adapted animal seems to have a slightly higher background perfusate activity level than the dark-adapted animal, neither animal shows any change in level throughout the perfusion period.

Fig. 8.10 summarizes the changes in rate of release of radioactivity into the perfusate which occurred in each experimental group. Expressing this release in terms of millimicromoles of H3-DA is justified on the basis of the radiochromatography results described below. Although the release of H3-DA is clearly different in the various experimental groups, the total amount of radioactivity released during the release phase is essentially identical in all groups as shown in Fig. 8.11. This total release, or area under each

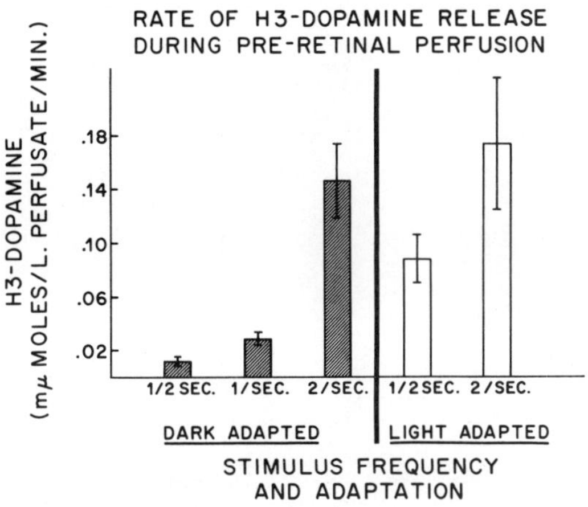

Fig. 8.10. Summary of rate of H3-DA release (slope of fitted line during rising portion of release curve) for animals in Groups I to V, Figs. 8.7 and 8.8.

release curve (Figs. 8.7 and 8.8), is fixed and is related presumably to the amount of exogenously administered H3-DA the uptake system of the preparation is capable of retaining.

Finally, one animal in each experimental group underwent bilateral optic nerve section prior to perfusion. The perfusion results in these animals were essentially identical to the results from the other animals in each respective group.

Radiochromatography of the pooled perfusates obtained during the release phases of all 15 experiments is demonstrated in Fig. 8.12. Sixty-six per cent of the radioactivity in the pooled perfusates migrated chromatographically with authentic dopamine. There was a small amount of activity associated with norepinephrine (11 per cent) but almost none with any other of the dopamine metabolites tested.

Autoradiography. Autoradiographs of the retina following the "washout phase" of preretinal perfusion with H3-dopamine revealed a striking band of radioactivity precisely at the junction of the inner nuclear and inner plexiform layers (Fig. 8.13). Discrete activity was apparent in this location with as little as one day of exposure of the nuclear emulsion to the section.

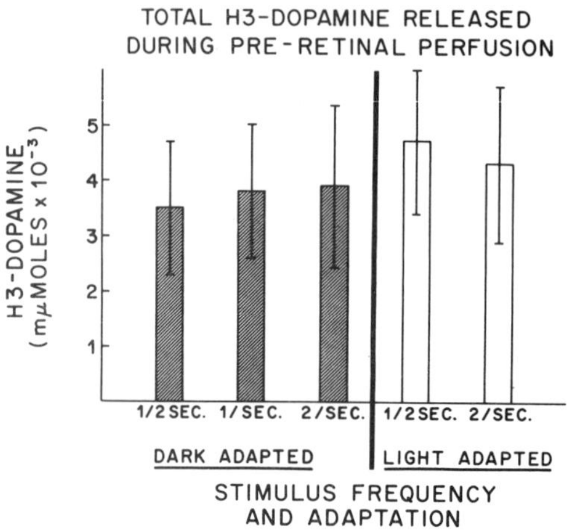

Fig. 8.11. Total radioactivity (area under release curve) in perfusate during "release phase" of preretinal perfusion for animals in Groups I to V, Figs. 8.7 and 8.8.

The emulsion overlying the sections tended to obscure detail and to induce an excessively pink color to the over-all section. Fig. 8.14 shows a section from the same experimental eye as those shown in the other figures, but in this case no nuclear emulsion was applied. It demonstrates satisfactory tissue fixation with clear anatomic detail and lack of the general blur induced by the emulsion. The junctional area (arrow) of radioactivity localization is shown at similar power for comparison in Fig. 8.15. Diffuse activity is present to greatest extent in the inner plexiform layer, next in the inner nuclear layer, and least in the outer plexiform and outer nuclear layers.

Fig. 8.16 from an area of dense activity, shows a single cell from the junctional region which heavily concentrates the radioactive label. Arrows indicate the outline of this cell body.

Occasional single cells with specific localization of radioactivity were seen in the ganglion cell layer. Fig. 8.17 demonstrates such a cell with almost no surrounding background activity. Neuronal processes containing label could not be seen associated with these cells.

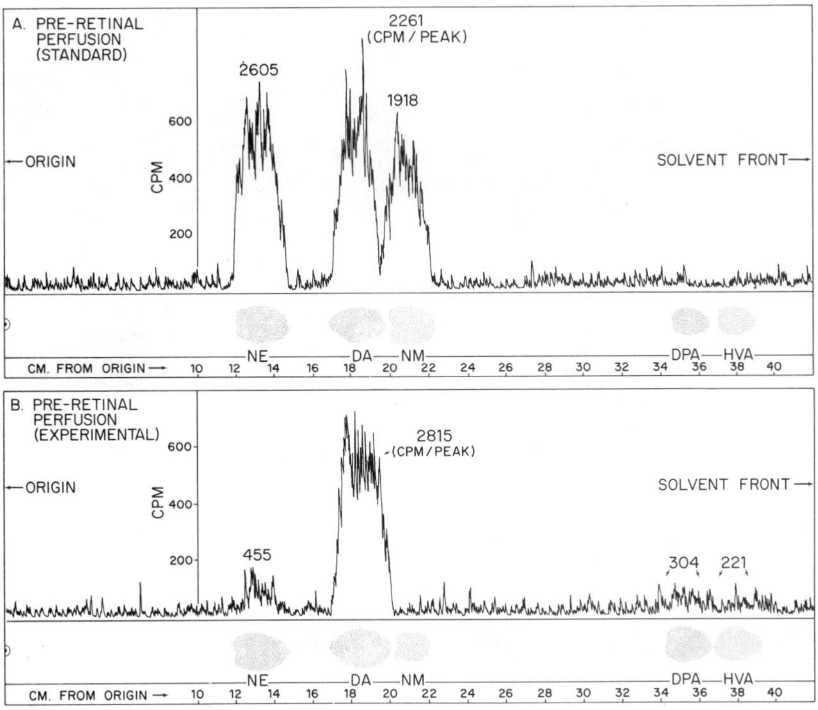

Fig. 8.12. Radiochromatography of pooled perfusates obtained during "release phase" of preretinal perfusion in all animals of Groups I to V. (A) Tracing of standard chromatogram; (B) tracing of experimental chromatogram of pooled perfusates run simultaneously with standard. (SCAN) Recorder output from radiochromatogram scanner; (STRIP) chromatogram strip; spots are tracings of actual spots on chromatogram strips; (CPM) counts per minute; (NE) norepinephrine; (DA) dopamine; (NM) normetanephrine; (DPA) dihydroxyphenylacetic acid, and (HVA) homovanillic acid. Number above peak indicates area under peak or CPM per peak.

Retinal autoradiographs following carotid infusion of H3-catecholamines showed very little discrete localization of activity even with as much as three months of exposure to the emulsion. This was in contradistinction to the choroid in the same sections in which specific neuronal localization of radioactivity was readily seen.

DISCUSSION

In a flush of enthusiasm which followed rapid advances in the area of chemical neurotransmission, neuropharmacologists established a group of fairly rigid criteria considered necessary for the identification of transmitters (Curtis, 1961, and McLennan, 1963) (Table 8.1). Subsequent developments proceeded more slowly, particularly as investigators turned their attention toward the central nervous system. The criterion makers had established guidelines which, from an experimental viewpoint, were extremely difficult to apply to studies of central nervous system (CNS) synapses. Werman (1966) has discussed the inaccessibility of central synapses and has suggested that "slavish" adherence to previous criteria and experimental techniques may hinder our understanding of CNS transmitter processes.

The retina, however, is uniquely more accessible to experimentation than other parts of the CNS. This accessibility, as demonstrated in the present chapter, makes it possible to apply classical neurotransmission criteria to studies of retinal synaptology. The preretinal perfusion technique described here allows an uptake and release experiment on CNS tissue without any disorganization of the highly organized histoanatomy of that tissue. The emphasis on the function of retinal dopamine also simplifies matters, as this substance is so specifically localized to a very limited area and group of cells within the retina (Ehinger, 1966; Laties and Jacobowitz, 1966 a and b; Sano, Yoshikawa and Konishi, 1968; Ehinger, Falck and Laties, 1969; Ehinger and Falck, 1969). Uptake and release measurements of dopamine made across the retina as a whole apply presumably specifically to the dopamine-containing retinal neurons, and only to these neurons (Whitby, Axelrod and Weil-Malherbe, 1961; Iversen, 1967).

There is now evidence available supporting all five classic criteria (Table 8.1) for the establishment of the neurotransmitter role of retinal dopamine.

Criterion 1: The Presence of Dopamine in Retinal Neurons

The histochemical studies of dopamine-containing retinal neurons (Ehinger, 1966; Laties and Jacobowitz, 1966 a and b; Sano, Yoshikawa and Konishi, 1968; Ehinger, Falck and Laties, 1969; Ehinger and Falck, 1969), and the chemical

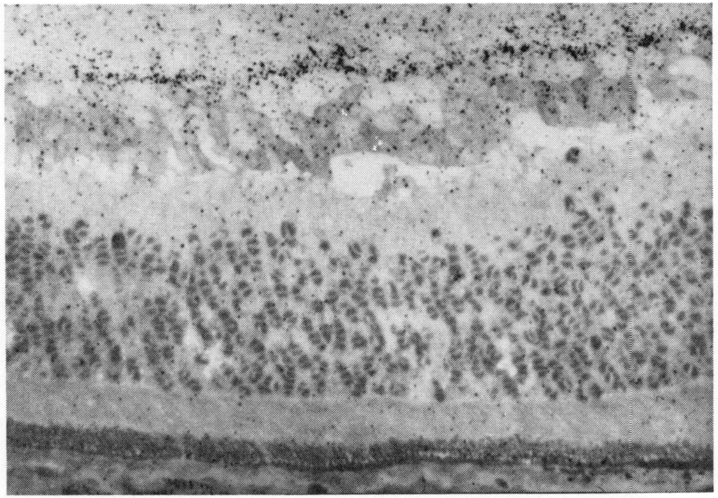

Fig. 8.13. Autoradiograph of cat retina following washout phase of preretinal perfusion with H3-dopamine, three-week exposure. Note band of silver grains at junction of inner nuclear and inner plexiform layers. (Toluidine blue-pyronin B, Ilford K-5 emulsion. Original magnification x I30.).

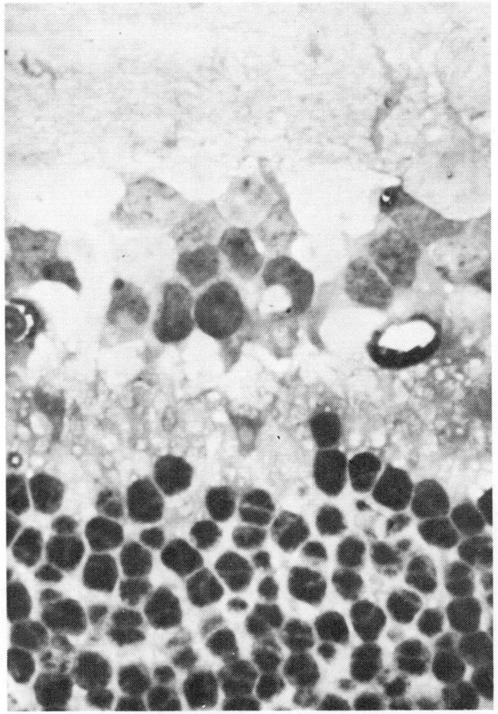

Fig. 8.14. Section of same retina as shown in other figures without overlying nuclear emulsion. (Toluidine blue-pyronin B. Original magnification x 320).

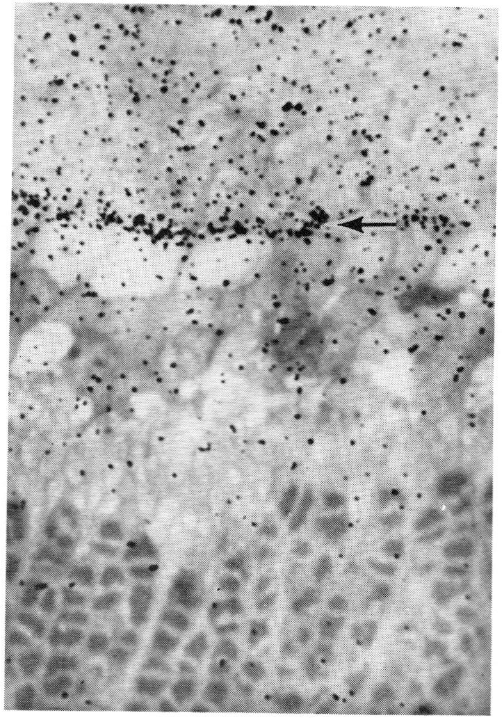

Fig. 8.15. High-power autoradiograph showing band of activity at junction of inner nuclear and inner plexiform layers as in Fig. 8.13, three-week exposure. (Toluidine blue-pyronin B, Ilford K-5 emulsion. Original magnification x 320).

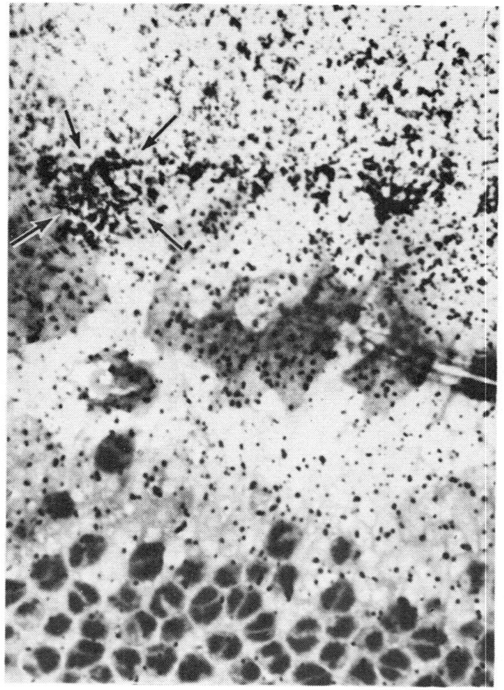

Fig. 8.16. High-power autoradiograph showing labeled cell (arrows) within densely labeled band of activity at junction of inner nuclear and inner plexiform layers, four-week exposure. This is probably the *dopaminergic junctional cell* (see text and Fig. 8.19). (*Toluidine blue-pyronin B*, Ilford K-5 emulsion. Original magnification x 400).

determinations of Haggendal and Malmfors (1965), and Nichols and co-workers (Nichols et al., 1967) have already been enumerated. It is well established that the retinal dopamine-containing neurons are independent of the sympathetic system of the eye, and that they are similar in location and morphology to retinal amacrine cells (Carlsson, 1966; Sano, Yoshikawa and Konishi, 1968; Ehinger, Falck and Laties, 1969; Ehinger and Falck, 1969).

That retinal H3-DA retention after carotid infusion is not altered by cervical ganglionectomy (Figs. 8.1 and 8.2), is further evidence that retinal dopamine-containing neurons are independent of ocular sympathetics.

Evidence for storage of exogenously administered dopamine in these same retinal neurons is presented in the autoradiographic data reported here.

As shown in Figs. 8.13 to 8.17, autoradiographic localization of H3-dopamine was very discrete and corresponded exactly to the distribution of neurons which are known to contain endogenous dopamine. The band of localized activity at the junction of the inner nuclear and inner plexiform layers (Figs. 8.13 and 8.15) corresponds to a fluorescent band seen by the histochemical technique of Falck and Owman (1965) in a wide variety of species (Nichols, Jacobowitz and Hottenstein, 1967; Ehinger, 1966; Laties and Jacobowitz, 1966 a and b; Sano, Yoshikawa and Konishi, 1968; Ehinger, Falck and Laties, 1969; Ehinger and Falck, 1969). The single cell which is heavily laden with activity in Fig. 8.16 probably corresponds to similar single fluorescent cells seen within the band of fluorescent fibers at the junction of the inner nuclear and inner plexiform layers (Nichols, Jacobowitz and Hottenstein, 1967; Ehinger, 1966; Laties and Jacobowitz, 1966 a and b; Sano, Yoshikawa and Konishi, 1968; Ehinger, Falck and Laties, 1969; Ehinger and Falck, 1969). Such cells are similar to amacrine cells, but in most species they comprise only about ten per cent of these cells (Ehinger, 1966; Laties and Jacobowitz, 1966 a and b). Recently, Ehinger and Falck (1969) have proposed the term "adrenergic junctional cells" to describe these.

The occasional cell in the ganglion cell layer which concentrates tritiated dopamine following preretinal perfusion (Fig. 8.17) probably corresponds to the "alloganglion cells" described by Ehinger (1966). In virtually all species, occasional cells in the ganglion cell layer fluoresce for the presence of catecholamines. Connections of these have not been observed, and perhaps they represent ectopic cells from the junctional region. In any case, their endogenous catecholamine content suggests a capacity for exogenous catecholamine uptake and storage, and this is supported by the autoradiographic findings exemplified by Fig. 8.17. Finally, the relatively dense though diffuse activity of the inner plexiform region (Fig. 8.15) suggests the possibility of specific uptake and storage in this region. Catecholamine-containing fibers in this region have been called "eremite" fibers by Ehinger (1966), and they may be responsible for the activity observed.

Criterion 2: Mechanism for Synthesis and Degradation of Dopamine in Retinal Neurons

The presence of dopamine in the retina does not imply necessarily the presence of mechanisms for its synthesis in the same tissue, for it may be transferred there from other synthetic sites. On the other hand, it is known that dopamine passes the blood-brain barrier very poorly (Fuxe and Hillarp, 1964), and its presence in brain implies, therefore, its synthesis in brain. If the same is true of the blood-retinal barrier, then dopamine's presence in the retina would imply its synthesis there as well. Our autoradiographic observations (Kramer, Potts and Mangnall, 1971) indicate far more efficient localization of H3-DA in retinal neurons by preretinal perfusion than by carotid infusion. This suggests that the blood-retinal barrier tends to exclude dopamine, and endogenous retinal dopamine is synthesized locally by the neurons in which it is observed.

Radiochromatography of the retinal extract following carotid infusion of H3-DA (Fig. 8.3) reveals the presence of significant amounts of known metabolites of dopamine: norepinephrine (product of dopamine-B-hydroxylase), dihydroxyphenylacetic acid (product of monoamine oxidase), and homovanillic acid (product of monoamine oxidase and catechol-O-methyl transferase) (Iversen, 1967). The implication is clear that these degradative enzymes occur intraretinally. As little or no norepinephrine is present in the retina (Haggendal and Malmfors, 1965; Nichols, Jacobowitz and Hottenstein, 1967), it is not surprising that there is little or no capacity for its breakdown present, and no normetanephrine is found in the extract. This is in contradistinction to tissues such as the iris and ciliary body which contain norepinephrine and which form normetanephrine from exogenously administered norepinephrine (Kramer and Potts, 1969 a and b).

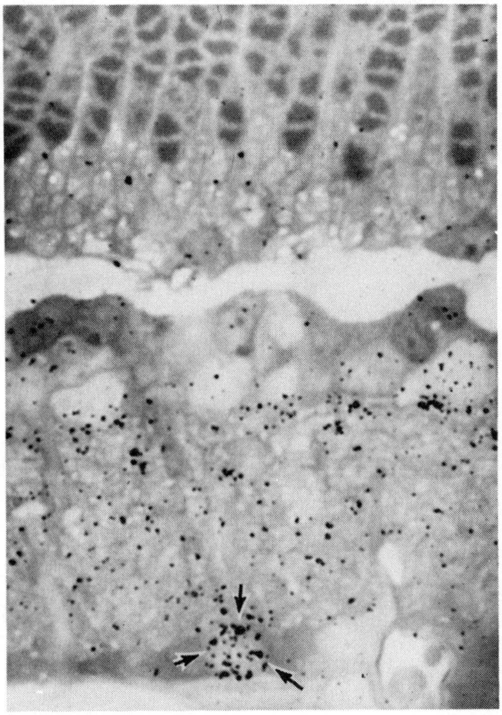

Fig. 8.17. High-power autoradiograph showing labeled cell (arrow) within ganglion cell layer, one-week exposure. (Toluidine blue-pyronin B, Ilford K-5 emulsion. Original magnification x 320.).

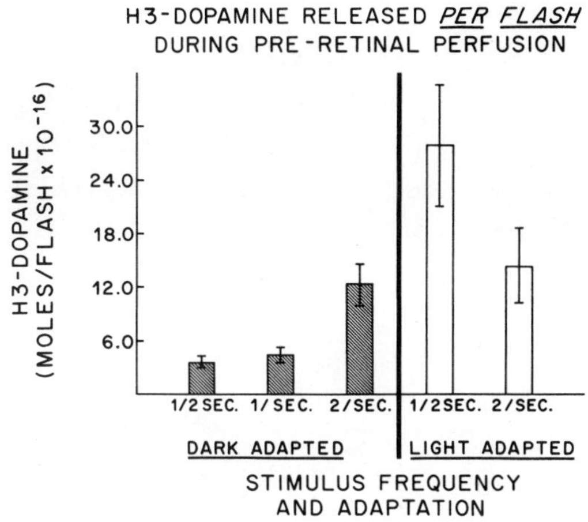

Fig. 8.18. Release of H3-DA for each flash during rising portion of release curve for animals in Groups I to V, Figs. 8.7 and 8.8.

Criterion 3: Release of Dopamine when Retinal Neurons are Stimulated

The preretinal perfusion experiments described in this chapter demonstrate release of H3-DA from the retina; this release is induced by a flashing light stimulus and does not occur to a detectable extent without such a stimulus. The possibility that the observed effects are actually mediated via other catecholamine-containing tissues, such as those of the uveal tract, is eliminated by the experiments in which bilateral optic nerve section was done without a change in results. Any uveal release phenomenon induced by light would have to be mediated by the central nervous system, and optic nerve section precludes such mediation. Retinal neurons are the only ones which still have neural connection to the photoreceptors following bilateral section of the optic nerves.

At least in the dark-adapted state, the rate of H3-DA release from the retina increases nonlinearly with increasing stimulus rates (Figs. 8.7 and 8.10). The same data expressed in terms of amount of H3-DA released for each stimulus flash during the ascending limb of the release curve (Figs. 8.7 and 8.8) are shown in Fig. 8.18. In the dark-adapted animals, with increasing flash rate, there is actually a progressive increase in the amount of H3-DA released for each flash. Increasing the rate of a flickering stimulus is well-known to decrease the over-all level of retinal sensitivity (Arden, Granit and Ponte, 1960; Dowling, 1963). If increasing the rate of such a stimulus also increases the amount of H3-DA released for each stimulus as noted above, it is consistent to suppose that the dopamine may at least partially mediate the decreased retinal sensitivity--perhaps by acting as an inhibitory neurotransmitter. More direct evidence on the inhibitory aspects of retinal dopamine function will be presented elsewhere (Kramer, Potts and Buffum, in preparation).

In the light-adapted state, the change in H3-DA release with a change in stimulus rate is less clear (Fig. 8.8). Under these conditions, even a very slow stimulus seems to drive the dopamine-releasing mechanism at a high rate. Perhaps the background light induces a further reduction in retinal sensitivity which, again, is partially mediated by dopaminergic inhibitory neurotransmission. The unexplained fact remains, however, that no measurable release occurs with or without background illumination unless a flashing stimulus is introduced (Fig. 8.9).

The data on H3-DA release obtained in this study are actually data on radioactivity release. The radiochromatography done on pooled pefusates (Fig. 8.12) establishes that the great majority of this radioactivity is in fact H3-DA. There is no evidence to suggest a transmitter role for any other substance in the present study.

Criterion 4: Discharge (or Inhibition) of Postsynaptic Neuron by the Direct Application of Dopamine

Our studies offer no evidence in support of this criterion. Straschill and Perwein (1969), however, have shown an inhibition in retinal ganglion-cell firing rate induced by iontophoretic application of dopamine. In general, they found that dopamine tended to depress excitatory and enhance inhibitory phenomena. In isolated retinal preparations, Ames and Pollen (1969) also found inhibitory effects of dopamine.

Hedden and Dowling (1975) have recently reported both depolarizing and hyperpolarizing effects of applied dopamine on horizontal cells in teleost retinas. They applied dopamine in solution by an atomizer technique and observed the two types of responses in different horizontal cells.

Criterion 5: Pharmacologic "Blockers" of Dopamine Should Block Transmission Effects

To investigate the thesis that retinal dopamine is an inhibitory neurotransmitter which partially mediates retinal sensitivity level, we studied the effects of systemic reserpine administration on electroretinographic flicker suppression (Kramer, Potts and Buffum, in preparation). Reserpine was given in systemic doses which could be expected to deplete retinal dopamine (Haggendal and Malmfors, 1965), and a decrease in ERG flicker suppression effect was found.

Unfortunately, this work has been plagued by a massive systemic effect on the animals of the reserpinizing dose required, and the results have yet to be confirmed by other more selective routes of reserpine administration or by other means of dopamine blockade. For this reason, detailed methodology and results are not presented, but the following preliminary impressions can be outlined.

After massive systemic reserpinization which reduced retinal dopamine levels essentially to zero, there was reduction or loss of the phenomenon known as electroretinographic flicker suppression. This inhibitory depression of the ERG b-wave in the slowly flickering electroretinogram tended to disappear when the retina was depleted of dopamine. The phenomenon recovered after systemic administration of DOPA, and the recovery was largely prevented by DOPA-decarboxylase inhibition. These observations are undergoing further study utilizing different pharmacologic inhibitors and blockers and different routes of administration.

It can also be added in the context of this review that another preparation for the study of retinal uptake and release of dopamine is being developed and has not yet been reported. This involves a preretinal perfusion, similar to the one described here, which is different in the sense that the eye is left intact, the intraocular pressure is maintained, and the vitreous cavity is isolated and perfused without destructive surgery to the anterior portion of the experimental eye. The newer clinical tools for vitreous surgery and vitrectomy are utilized in a preparatory operation, which is followed some weeks later by the experimental preparation and procedures.

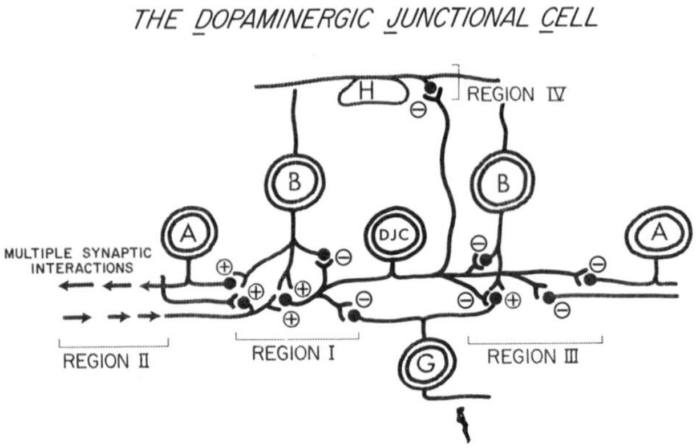

Fig. 8.19. Schematic conception of the dopaminergic junctional cell (DJC) (see text and Fig. 8.16). H = horizontal cell, B = bipolar cells, A = amacrine cells, G = ganglion cell. Regions I, II, and III (see text).

What begins to emerge from evidence presented in papers cited in this report, and from the results detailed here, is the possibility that dopamine functions as a retinal neurotransmitter at the endings of a rather specific group of retinal cells (Kramer, 1971). It seems possible that the cells which Ehinger and Falck (1966 and 1969) have called adrenergic junctional cells are actually dopaminergic junctional cells with rather specific characteristics (Fig. 8.19). They are similar in morphology and location to retinal amacrine cells, though in number they comprise about ten per cent of these in most species. On chemical and histochemical grounds, they contain significant amounts of dopamine. They are capable of accumulating and storing dopamine and of releasing it as a consequence of light stimulation of the retina. They have wide-ranging, horizontally oriented fibers which are among the longest of any retinal cells, and they may have inhibitory effects (Fig. 8.7, Region I). They may have multiple synaptic interactions with a variety of retinal cell types (Region II), and they may have small vertically oriented fibers extending back through the inner nuclear layer toward the horizontal cells (Region III). To date, these latter retrograde fibers have been identified as dopamine containing fibers only in teleost fish and New World monkeys.

In addition, Boycott and co-workers (Boycott et al., 1971) have reported amacrine-like cells, especially in the cat retina, which send distinct fibers vertically toward the outer plexiform layer. These comprise approximately ten per cent of the cat amacrine cells, the same number which tend to stain for the presence of dopamine. The retrograde fibers extending from the inner plexiform layer to the outer plexiform, horizontal cell layer are of particular interest in the light of the work mentioned earlier in which Hedden and Dowling (1975) reported dopamine effects on horizontal cell discharge. The intriguing possibility of a feedback inhibitory or excitatory system traversing the middle, bipolar portion of the retina, is raised by these observations. This is of particular interest because of the dearth of information which has been developed which might give any clue to the function of these baffling dopamine-containing retinal cells. The evidence of dopamine synthesis, uptake, storage, and release by these cells has not been followed by firm evidence of their electrophysiologic or neurophysiologic function.

This has been particularly frustrating, because the relative accessibility of the retina and of this particular population of cells led us to believe that this might be an exceptionally useful handle on basic retinal neuropharmacologic or neurophysiologic mechanisms.

Finally, the possibility must be raised, though it is not treated in detail here, that a major function of retinal dopamine involves metabolic control systems related to cyclic AMP and adenylcyclase. A burgeoning literature is appearing which is suggestive of major effects of retinal dopamine in this system (Brown and Makman, 1973; Atterwill and Neal, 1973; ch. 9 of this book).

In any case it is to be hoped that painstaking and careful study of these retinal cells will prove more fruitful in the future, or at least that the experimental methodology evolved for their study will prove useful in the investigation of other aspects of retinal neuropharmacology.

ACKNOWLEDGEMENTS

I wish to express my sincere gratitude to Albert Potts, Alfred Heller, J. Terry Ernest, Joel Pokorny, Vivian Smith, Yvonne Magnall, and David Buffum who participated in this work at the University of Chicago. This work was supported in part by Research Grant number 5033-01 from the Veterans Administration Hospital and in part by USPHS Research Grants numbers EY-01373, EY-0065, EY-00416 and EY-47078-01.

I also wish to acknowledge with thanks Investigative Ophthalmology's kind permission to reprint the figures and material presented here. Reprint requests to: Steven G. Kramer, M.D., Ph.D., Department of Ophthalmology, University of California Medical Center, San Francisco, California 94143. (Room 490-U).

REFERENCES

Ames A. and Pollen D.A. (1969) Neurotransmission in central nervous tissue - a study of isolated rabbit retina. J. Neurophysiol. 32, 424

Arden G., Granit R. and Ponte F. (1960) Phase of suppression following each retinal b-wave in flicker. J. Neurophysiol. 23, 305

Atterwill C.K. and Neal M.J. (June 1973) The subcellular distribution of 14C-Gamma-Aminobutyric Acid Gaba and 3H-Dopamine in the rabbit retina. Br. J. Pharmacol. 48 (2), 355-356

Bertler A., Carlsson A. and Rosengren E. (1958) A method for the fluorimetric determination of adrenaline and noradrenaline in tissues. Acta Physiol. Scand. 44, 273

Boycott B., Dowling J., Fisher S., Kolb H. and Laties A.M. (April 30, 1971) A new amacrine cell in the vertebrate retina. Presented at the Spring National Meeting of the Association for Research in Vision and Ophthalmology

Brown J.H. and Makman M.H. (August 1973) Influence of neuroleptic drugs and apomorphine on dopamine-sensitive adenylate cyclase of retina. J. Neurochem. 21 (2), 477-9

Carlsson A. (1966) Pharmacological depletion of catecholamine stores. Pharmacol. Rev. 18, 541

Curtis D.R. (1961) The identification of mammalian inhibitory transmitters. In: Florey E., ed.: Nervous Inhibition, Proceedings of the Second Friday Harbor Symposium, New York, Pergamon Press, Inc., p.342

Dowling J.E. (1963) Neural and photochemical mechanisms of visual adaptation in the rat. J. Gen. Physiol. 46, 1287

Ehinger B. (1966) Distribution of adrenergic nerves in the eye and some related structures in the cat. Acta Physiol. Scand. 66, 123

Ehinger B., Falck B. and Laties A.M. (1969) Adrenergic neurons in teleost retina. Z. Zellforsch., 97, 285

Ehinger B. and Falck B. (1969) Morphological and pharmacohistochemical characteristics of adrenergic retinal neurons of some mammals. Graefe. Arch. Klin. Exp. Ophthal. 178, 295

Falck B. and Owman C. (1965) A detailed methodological description of the fluorescence method for the cellular demonstration of biogenic monoamines. Acta Universitatis Lundensis, Section II, No. 7

Fleming R.M., Clark W.G., Fenster E.D. and Town J.C. (1965) Single extraction method for the simultaneous fluorometric determination of serotonin, and norepinephrine in brain. Anal. Chem. 37, 692

Fuxe K. and Hillarp N.A. (1964) Uptake of L-dopa and noradrenaline by central catecholamine neurons. Life Sci. 3, 1403
Goldbaum L.R. and Kazyak L. (1956) Identification of alkaloids and other basic drugs by paper partition chromatography. Anal. Chem. 28, 1289
Haggendal J. and Malmfors T. (1965) Identification and cellular localization of the catecholamines in the retina and the choroid of the rabbit. Acta Physiol. Scand. 64, 58
Haggendal J. (1967) An improved method for the fluorimetric determination of small amounts of adrenaline and noradrenaline in plasma and tissues. Acta Physiol. Scand. 57, 242
Halushka P.V. (1967) Studies on the distribution, metabolism, and mechanism of action of dopamine (Doctoral dissertation). Chicago, The University of Chicago, p. 14
Halushka P.V. and Hoffmann P.C. (1968) Does tetrahydropapaveroline contribute to the cardiovascular actions of dopamine? Biochem. Pharmacol. 17, 1873
Hedden W.L. and Dowling J.E. (1975) Dopamine effects on horizontal cells in the goldfish retina. Presented at the Association for Research in Vision and Ophthalmology Meeting, Sarasota, Florida, Apr. 28 - May 2
Iversen L.L. (1967) The metabolic degradation of catecholamines. In: The Uptake and Storage of Noradrenaline in Sympathetic Nerves. Cambridge, Cambridge University Press, p. 62
Iversen L.L. (1967) The uptake of catecholamines by sympathetic nerves. In: The Uptake and Storage of Noradrenaline in Sympathetic Nerves. Cambridge, Cambridge University Press, p. 108
Kasner D. (1968) Vitrectomy: A new approach to the management of vitreous. Highlights Ophthal. 11, 304
Kramer S.G. and Potts A.M. (1969) Iris uptake of catecholamines in experimental Horner's syndrome. Amer. J. Ophthal. 67, 705
Kramer S.G. and Potts A.M. (1969) Intraocular pressure and ciliary body norepinephrine uptake in experimental Horner's syndrome. Amer. J. Ophthal. 68, 1076
Kramer S.G. (1971) Dopamine: a retinal neurotransmitter. I. Retinal uptake, storage, and light-stimulated release of H3-dopamine in vivo. Invest. Ophth. 10, 438-452
Kramer S.G., Potts A.M. and Mangnall Y. (1971) Dopamine: a retinal neurotransmitter. II. Autoradiographic localization of H3-dopamine in the retina. Invest. Ophth. 10, 617
Kramer S.G., Potts A.M. and Buffum D. (in preparation) Dopamine: a retinal neurotransmitter. III. Reserpine-induced inhibition of electroretinographic flicker suppression.
Krill A.E., Potts A.M. and Johanson C. (1971) Chloroquine retinopathy. Investigation of discrepancy between dark adaptation and electroretinographic findings in advanced stages. Amer. J. Ophthal. 71, 530
Laties A.M. and Jacobowitz D. (1966) Histochemical studies of monoamine-containing cells in the monkey retina. J. Histochem. Cytochem. 14, 823
Laties A.M. and Jacobowitz D. (1966) A comparative study of the autonomic innervation of the eye in monkey, cat, and rabbit. Anat. Rec. 156, 383
McLennan H. (1963) The concept of chemical transmission. In: Synaptic Transmission, Philadelphia, W.B. Saunders, p. 23
Nichols C.W., Jacobowitz D. and Hottenstein M. (1967) The influence of light and dark on the catecholamine content of the retina and choroid. Invest. Ophthal. 6, 642
Sano Y., Yoshikawa H. and Konishi M (1968) Fluorescence microscopic observations on the dog retina. Arch. Hist. Jap. 30, 75
Straschill M. and Perwein J. (1969) The inhibition of retinal ganglion cells by catecholamines and gamma-aminobutyric acid. Pflügers Arch. 312, 45

Werman R. (1966) Criteria for identification of a central nervous system transmitter. Comp. Biochem. Physiol. 18, 745

Whitby L.G., Axelrod J. and Weil-Malherbe H. (1961) The fate of H^3-norepinephrine in animals. J. Pharmacol. Exp. Therap. 132, 193

CHAPTER 9

CHARACTERIZATION OF CATECHOLAMINE RECEPTORS IN RAT RETINA

J.S. Wassenaar* and J. Korf[x]

*Dept. of Neurophysiology and [x]Inst. of Biological Psychiatry

University of Groningen, Groningen, The Netherlands

INTRODUCTION

This chapter will deal mainly with the possible role of catecholamines and their relationship with cyclic adenosine monophosphate (cAMP) in the neuronal network of the retina (Wassenaar et al., 1975). In the first three sections data from different disciplines will be presented to offer a background against which our experimental data described in the next four sections will be considered.

On the basis of embryological arguments the retina has to be considered as part of the central nervous system (see for review: Duke Elder and Cook, 1963). Thus some principles underlying the function of the retinal network can be derived from research on other brain structures (see e.g. Shepherd, 1974). On the other hand the retina also differs from the brain in several respects. The retina contains a sensory (photoreceptor layer) as well as an information processing structure (retinal network) (Dowling and Werblin, 1969; Bonting, this book, chapter 1). The electrical characteristics of retinal cells often differ from those of spike-generating neurons of the central nervous system. The slow onset and long-lasting activity of the horizontal and bipolar cells are rather similar to that of the photoreceptor cells. Amacrine cells, however, do show spike-like discharges upon illumination of the retina, while the large ganglion cells respond like ordinary neurons (Werblin and Dowling, 1969). For a detailed survey describing the sequence of events from photoreceptor to ganglion cell the reader is referred to Werblin (1974) and to the introductory chapter by Bonting in this book.

CATECHOLAMINES

Our studies are concerned with the influence of catecholamines on the levels of cyclic nucleotides in the retina. Our current knowledge on the localization of catecholamines in the retina is derived from the application of a variety of techniques: light- and electronmicroscopy (Stell, 1972; Dubin, 1974), histofluorescence (Falck et al., 1962; Malmfors, 1963) and autoradiography (Kramer et al., 1971), electrophysiological, neurochemical and neuropharmacological approaches (Ames and Pollen, 1969; Straschill and Perwein, 1969; Kramer, 1971).

Localization by histofluorescence and autoradiographic techniques

So far the histofluorescence method has been the most reliable technique for investigating the localization of catecholamines in the retina (Falck et al., 1962; Malmfors, 1963). Catecholamines, of which dopamine (DA) seems to be the main representative, have been found in the retina of many vertebrate species (Häggendal and Malmfors, 1965; Nichols et al., 1967; Ehinger and Falck, 1971; reviews: Graham, 1974; and Ehinger, this book, chapter 7).

Cells and cell extensions of the inner nuclear and inner synaptic layers of the retina appear to concentrate the largest part of the amines. Kramer et al. (1971) have used an autoradiographic technique to localize exogenously applied ^{3}H-DA. The distribution of this substance in the retina coincides perfectly with the distribution of catecholamine fluorescence.

Electrophysiological studies

To obtain more information about the physiological role of catecholamines in the retina, several investigators have studied the bioelectrical properties of retinal cells in the absence and presence of catecholamines. Straschill and Perwein (1969) showed that cat retinal ganglion cells decreased their firing frequency after iontophoretic application of DA and noradrenaline (NA), suggesting an inhibitory action of these amines. Ames and Pollen (1969) perfused rabbit retinae *in vitro* and measured firing rates of retinal ganglion cells in the absence or presence of catecholamines and of related compounds in combination with discrete light stimuli. DA and NA were found to increase the activity of OFF-cells and to decrease that of ON-cells and of ON-OFF-cells. Despite the use of α- and β-adrenergic antagonists, the authors were unable to characterize the adrenergic synapses involved in terms of DA- or NA-receptors.

Kramer has developed a preretinal perfusion technique, in which the cat eye ball *in situ* is transformed into a perfusion chamber (Kramer, 1971; Kramer et al., 1971). With this technique it is found that cat retinae, previously labeled with ^{3}H-dopamine, release this amine after stimulation with light flashes. The release is dependent on the flash frequency. Cat retinae, labeled with ^{3}H-dopamine and kept "silent" in a dark or light adapted state, do not release dopamine. For more detailed information about the action of catecholamines on bioelectrical phenomena in the retinal network we refer to Kramer (this book, chapter 8).

POTASSIUM IONS AND NERVOUS FUNCTION

Potassium ions appear to be involved in the regulation of several physiological functions in the nervous system:

1) Potassium ions govern the distribution of water and electrolytes in brain tissue. Moreover, increased potassium levels in the medium or plasma cause a considerable increase of the intracellular water and electrolyte contents *in vitro* (Hertz, 1968; Franck, 1970; Lund-Andersen and Hertz, 1970; Hertz, 1973) as well as *in vivo* (Bourke, 1969; Bourke et al., 1970).
2) Potassium ions enhance the oxygen consumption in those parts of the central nervous system, which already have a high oxygen uptake, viz. the cortex (Hertz, 1966 and 1968).
3) Potassium ions are, together with Na^+- and Cl^--ions, the main cations which maintain the bioelectric activity in nervous tissue (Eccles, 1964; Hertz, 1973).
4) Potassium fluxes across postsynaptic membranes of various structures are triggered by neurotransmitters, resulting in either hyperpolarization or depolarization of the membrane. This latter effect determines the excitatory or inhibitory properties of the neurotransmitter involved (Kerkut et al., 1969; Ascher, 1972).
5) Raised levels of potassium in the medium increase the synthesis of cAMP in incubated nervous tissue. For brain slices this has been demonstrated by several investigators (Huang et al., 1971; Huang and Daly, 1974; Ferrendelli, 1973). Roch and Kalix (1975) have reported comparable effects for incubated fragments of superior cervical ganglion. Similar increases in the cAMP level have been observed by Brown and Makman (1972) upon incubating retinae in the presence of 83 mM K^+. These effects have been ascribed to depolarization of membrane structures. Though depolarization is certainly evoked by elevated K^+ concentrations, the exact mechanism for K^+-induced cAMP-synthesis remains to be elucidated (Roch and Kalix, 1975).

The mechanism(s) by which potassium ions exert these various effects are still uncertain (see however: Hertz, 1973). Whether the K^+-induced cAMP-synthesis has a role in one or more of the other processes mentioned is also unclear. In our studies we have, therefore, compared the effects of K^+ ions with those of catecholamine-induced cAMP synthesis.

THE DOPAMINE SENSITIVE ADENYL CYCLASE SYSTEM IN THE RETINA

The relation between the release of neurotransmitters in nervous structures and the subsequent induction of cyclic nucleotide synthesis has been described already by Bonting (this book, chapter 1).

For the retina two separate adenyl cyclase systems have been described during the last five years. One is localized in the outer segments of the photoreceptors (Bitensky, 1973). This adenyl cyclase system has been reviewed by Goridis (this book, chapter 2).

The other adenyl cyclase system is localized in the neuronal network and is sensitive to DA and possibly to other catecholamines (Brown and Makman, 1972). Hence, it seems to be involved in certain synaptic processes of the retina. We shall deal with this "neuronal system" in the next sections of this chapter.

Comparing the retinal DA-sensitive adenyl cyclase system with systems of other organs, we arrive at two other structures which possess a DA-sensitive cyclase: the superior cervical sympathetic ganglion (McAfee, 1971; Cramer et al., 1973; Greengard et al., 1972), and the caudate nucleus (Kebabian et al., 1972; Mishra et al., 1974; Makman et al., 1975). From experiments with the superior cervical sympathetic ganglion of rabbits, Greengard et al. (1972) gathered evidence that DA induces changes in cAMP-levels in postsynaptic structures. Their concept of a DA-receptor coupled to an adenyl cyclase system could very well hold for the "neuronal" system of the retina as well.

Studies with specific drugs, which act on DA-receptors and which can be synergistic (apomorphine) or antagonistic (haloperidol and fluphenazine) have offered strong evidence for a DA-receptor coupled adenyl cyclase in the retina (Brown and Makman, 1972 and 1973; Makman et al., 1975; Bucher and

Schorderet, 1975).

From a comparative study Makman et al. (1975) conclude that the properties of the cyclase systems of the retina and the caudate nucleus are generally similar.

CHARACTERIZATION OF EXPERIMENTAL CONDITIONS

Our studies are mainly concerned with interactions between a potassium-stimulated cAMP synthetizing mechanism and catecholamine-sensitive cAMP synthetizing mechanisms.

Adult female Wistar albino rats (160-180 gr) and in a few cases pigmented rats (200 gr) were used throughout these studies. The retina is rapidly dissected from rat eyes removed immediately after decapitation. The retinae are preincubated for 40 min. in a balanced medium (according to Hertz, 1968) and subsequently incubated for 2 min. with a test substance dissolved in the incubation medium. During the entire incubation the medium is continuously gassed with a mixture of 95% O_2 and 5% CO_2. All incubations are performed at $37^{o}C$, and are stopped by homogenization of the retina in 50% acetic acid.

Further preparation of samples and determinations of cAMP are carried out according to Brown and Makman (1972). All agents used were of highest purity.

Histological examination of retinae, which are incubated for 42 min. and are immediately fixed and stained thereafter, shows no obvious histological abnormalities when compared with retinae fixed and stained immediately after dissection (Fig. 9.1).

In order to obtain reproducible DA-induced changes in cAMP levels, we find it necessary to incubate the retinal preparations in the presence of theophylline, an inhibitor of the cAMP-hydrolyzing enzyme phosphodiesterase. This is in accordance with the results of Brown and Makman (1972), and it is true for light adapted as well as for dark adapted retinae (Fig. 9.2). In

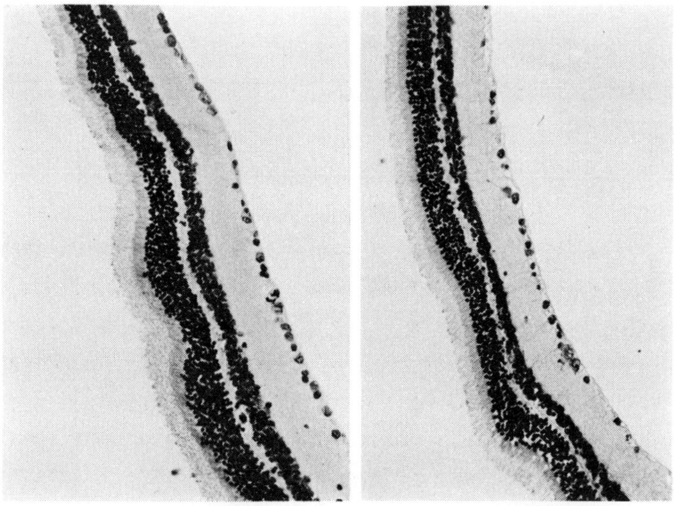

a b

Fig. 9.1. Histology of rat retina before and after incubation. a) immediately fixed after isolation (3 min.) following decapitation, b) fixed after 42 min. incubation. Fixation: Bouin d'Hollande.

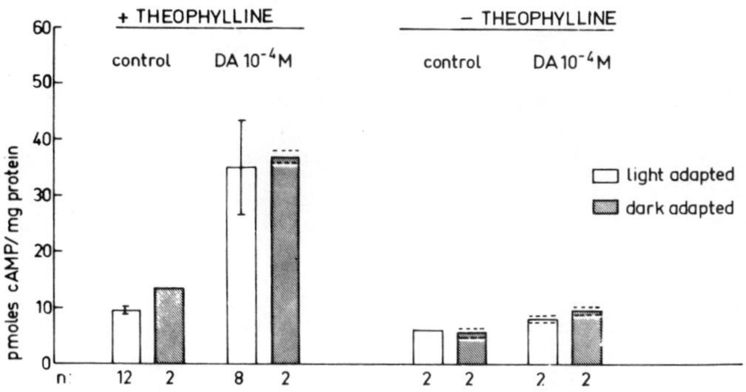

Fig. 9.2. Cyclic AMP levels in rat retina in the presence or absence of theophylline ($2x10^{-3}$ M) and of dopamine (DA; 10^{-4} M). Dark adapted: retina dissected in dim red light from dark adapted rats (16 hours complete darkness), incubations also performed in dim red light. Light adapted: dissection of retina from light adapted rats, incubations performed under normal light conditions.

all experiments we have used 2 mM theophylline. We have also established that the DA-induced cAMP levels of light- and dark-adapted retinae do not show gross differences (Fig. 9.3). This agrees with the finding of Kramer (1971) that "silent" retinae kept either in the dark or in the light do not release DA.

Comparison between cAMP levels of retinae of pigmented rats and albino rats, incubated in the absence and presence of DA, also reveals no differences. We have tested the DA-induced cAMP-synthesis in pigmented and in albino retina in the presence of haloperidol (HALO). This compound is a local anaesthetic, known to block DA-receptors. In 10^{-4} M concentration it appears to abolish the DA-induced cAMP-synthesis in pigmented as well as in albino retinae (Table 9.1). On the basis of these results further experiments have been carried out with albino rats.

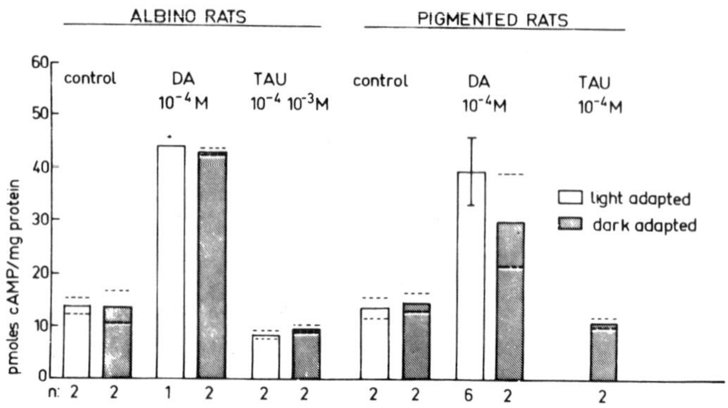

Fig. 9.3. Cyclic AMP levels in retina of albino and pigmented rats incubated in the presence or absence of dopamine (DA; 10^{-4} M) or taurine (Tau; 10^{-3} and 10^{-4} M). Incubations performed in dark and light adapted state (see legend Fig. 9.2).

Table 9.1. Cyclic AMP levels in retina of albino and pigmented rats in the presence of various agents

Agents	Retina	
	albino	pigmented
none	12; 15	12; 16
DA, 10^{-4} M	44	40
DA, 10^{-4} M + HALO, 10^{-4} M	10; 10	9; 8

Results are expressed in pmoles cAMP/mg protein.

In order to learn more about the specificity of the effects on the cAMP level in the retina a series of putative neurotransmitters, viz. taurine, glutamate, γ-amino butyric acid and NA in addition to DA, have been tested. Only DA and NA appear to be effective, both giving a 3-4 fold enhancement of the cAMP-level.

EFFECTS OF POTASSIUM IONS, OUABAIN, DOPAMINE AND NORADRENALINE

In our experiments with potassium we have used moderately elevated concentrations of this cation in order to avoid large water- and electrolyte shifts and extensive depolarization of retinal structures, thus maintaining relatively physiological conditions. Besides raised potassium levels we have used ouabain which depolarizes neuronal membranes by inhibiting the cation pump mechanism.

In one series of experiments we compared the effects of K^+ and ouabain with those obtained with DA and NA (Fig. 9.4). A clear stimulation of cAMP synthesis occurs during incubation with K^+-ions (30 mM), ouabain (10^{-4} M), DA (10^{-4} M) or NA (10^{-4} M). This is in accordance with the findings of Brown and Makman (1972). These effects have been further characterized by measuring time- and dose-dependency of the effect.

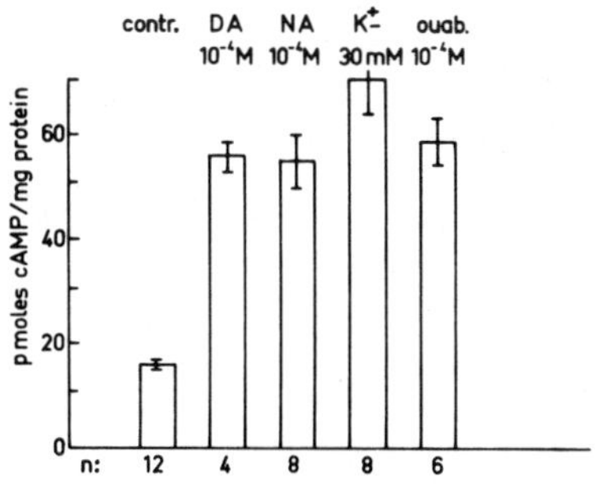

Fig. 9.4. Cyclic AMP levels in rat retina incubated in the presence of K^+-ions (30 mM), ouabain (10^{-4} M), noradrenaline (NA; 10^{-4} M) or dopamine (DA; 10^{-4} M). Control incubations in balanced medium containing 5 mM K^+. Number of experiments: 4-6. Vertical bars: 2x S.E.M.

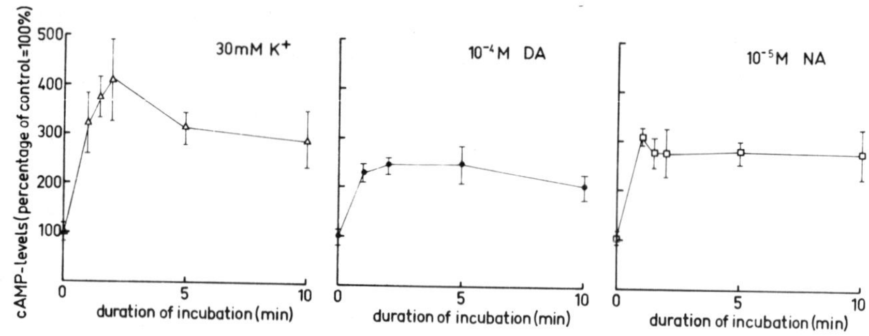

Fig. 9.5. Cyclic AMP levels in rat retina incubated with 30 mM K^+, 10^{-4} M NA or 10^{-4} M DA as a function of incubation time. Control values between 10-20 pmoles/mg protein; potassium concentration in control incubations: 5 mM; number of experiments for each point: 4. Vertical bars: 2x S.E.M.

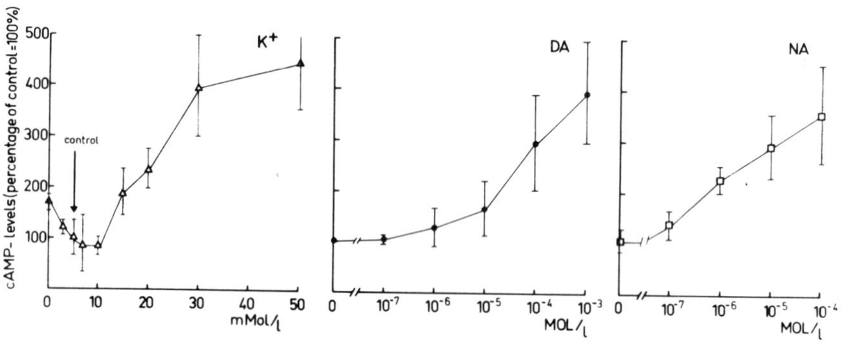

Fig. 9.6. Cyclic AMP levels in incubated rat retina as a function of K^+-, NA- and DA-concentrations. Control values between 15 and 24 pmoles/mg protein; potassium concentration in control incubations: 5 mM; number of experiments for each point: 4. Vertical bars: 2x S.E.M.

First, we have established the time-dependency for K^+, DA and NA. Fig. 9.5 indicates that maximal cAMP-levels are reached within 2 min. of incubation. This points to a rapid mechanism for cAMP-synthesis, which is sensitive to K^+-ions, DA and NA. Our dose-dependence studies (Fig. 9.6) reveal an interesting effect at potassium levels between zero and 10 mM. In this concentration range the cAMP-levels decrease with increasing potassium concentration, the lowest cAMP-level occurring at 5 mM K^+. At higher potassium concentrations (10-50 mM) the cAMP-levels increase to much higher values. Considering that preincubation of the retinae is performed in the normal balanced medium containing 5 mM K^+, there can have been no depolarizing action during the first three incubations with 0.3 and 5 mM K^+. At the two lower K^+-levels there may even have been some hyperpolarization. For DA and NA we have obtained dose-effect curves which show a somewhat higher responsiveness for NA than for DA (Fig. 9.6). These data do not allow us to decide whether these increases in cAMP-level are caused by a single cyclic AMP-synthetizing system or by more than one.

EFFECTS OF HALOPERIDOL AND FLUPHENAZINE ON THE RISES IN cAMP-LEVELS

We have tried to find out whether K^+ and ouabain exert their actions on the adenyl cyclase system by means of a specific trigger, which is similar to that utilized by DA and NA. For this purpose we have studied the effects of two neuroleptic drugs, haloperidol (HALO) and fluphenazine (FLU). The former has not only psycho-active, but also local anaesthetic properties. It has some antagonistic specificity for DA-receptors (Kebabian et al., 1972; Brown and Makman, 1973). The latter is a more powerful DA-receptor blocking agent.

First, we have studied the effects of haloperidol on the K^+-, ouabain-, DA- and NA-induced cAMP-responses (Table 9.2). Haloperidol (10^{-4} M) completely suppresses the increase in cAMP-level produced by K^+ and ouabain. Opposite effects are found when the cAMP-levels in the presence of DA and NA are measured. The DA-induced increase in cAMP-level is completely abolished in the presence of 10^{-4} M haloperidol, while the NA-induced rise in cAMP is doubled.

We can suggest two different explanations for the similar effects of the drug haloperidol on the action of K^+, ouabain and DA and for the different effect of haloperidol on the action of NA: the mediator hypothesis and the conformation hypothesis. In the mediator hypothesis the DA-, K^+- and ouabain-induced increases in cAMP-level would be evoked by a single mediator, which is not identical with the DA-receptor, but is interconnected with it. This mediator, localized in postsynaptic membranes, would activate one or more adenyl cyclase systems. It would be triggered by ouabain, K^+-ions and DA in different ways on

Table 9.2. Effects of high Potassium, Ouabain, Dopamine, Noradrenaline and Haloperidol on cyclic AMP-levels in rat retina

Agents		Haloperidol 10^{-4} M
none	18 ± 2 (12)	18 ± 1 (12)
K^+, 30 mM	72 ± 6 (8)	18 ± 1 (4)
ouabain, 10^{-4} M	59 ± 5 (6)	19 ± 1 (6)
DA, 10^{-4} M	56 ± 3 (4)	20 ± 3 (3)
NA, 10^{-4} M	55 ± 5 (8)	111 ± 8 (6)

Results are expressed in pmoles cAMP/mg protein.
Mean values ± S.E.M. are given with number of incubated retinae in parentheses.

the other side of the membrane. This postulated mediator would have a strong affinity for haloperidol. Binding of haloperidol to the mediator would disturb its coupling to the adenyl cyclase system(s), thereby abolishing the increase of cAMP by K^+, ouabain and DA. For NA another mediator-adenyl cyclase complex would exist, which is activated by haloperidol.

In the conformation hypothesis we would postulate that haloperidol changes the conformation of the membrane in view of its local anaesthetic activity. This change in membrane conformation would lead to inhibition of the adenyl cyclase system(s) which are susceptible to DA, K^+ or ouabain. This conformational change should lead then for noradrenaline to a facilitation of the NA-induced cAMP synthesis.

We have tried to distinguish between these hypotheses in two ways. We have used lower concentrations of haloperidol, so as to make changes in membrane conformation less likely, in combination with lower concentrations of NA, DA, K^+ and ouabain; in other experiments we have used the more powerful DA-receptor blocking agent fluphenazine (Table 9.3). Haloperidol still appears to decrease the K^+-induced cAMP-levels at 10^{-5} M, but not at 10^{-6} M. Both concentrations of haloperidol are ineffective with respect to the ouabain-induced cAMP-levels. Only DA-receptors seem to remain susceptible to a certain extent even for 10^{-6} M haloperidol, which supports the relative specificity of this

Table 9.3. Effects of high Potassium, Ouabain, Dopamine, Noradrenaline, Haloperidol and Fluphenazine on cAMP-levels in rat retina

Agents		Haloperidol		Fluphenazine
		10^{-5} M	10^{-6} M	10^{-6} M
none	19 ± 2 (5)	18 ± 2 (5)	19 ± 1 (5)	18 ± 1 (5)
K^+, 20 mM	46 ± 6 (4)	29 ± 5 (4)	52 ± 1 (4)	48 ± 4 (4)
ouabain, 10^{-5} M	30 ± 2 (4)	31 ± 1 (4)	35 ± 3 (3)	32 ± 2 (4)
DA, 10^{-5} M	39 ± 5 (4)	19 ± 3 (3)	32 ± 3 (4)	18 ± 1 (4)
NA, 10^{-5} M	44 ± 10 (3)			170 ± 16 (4)

Results are expressed in pmoles cAMP/mg protein.
Mean values ± S.E.M. are given with number of incubated retinae in parentheses.

drug for DA-receptors. Fluphenazine has no effect either on the K^+- or on the ouabain-induced cAMP-increase, but it has an inhibitory effect on the action of DA. However, it shows the same opposite effects on DA- and NA-induced increases of cAMP-levels as does haloperidol. It is our feeling that results obtained so far do not permit us to decide in favour of one of the two hypotheses.

ONE OR TWO CATECHOLAMINE RECEPTORS

The opposite effects of fluphenazine and haloperidol on the DA- and NA-induced cAMP-increases raise the question whether one receptor is involved with dual specificity, or whether two interacting receptors, one for NA and one for DA, exist. The different effects on the K^+-ouabain-induced cAMP-increases (Tables 9.2 and 9.3) might even suggest the existence of different binding sites for these two neuroleptics, but we feel that experiments with higher fluphenazine concentrations are needed before such a conclusion can be drawn. In order to obtain an impression of the sensitivity of the NA-induced cAMP-synthesis for fluphenazine, we have determined the effect of this drug at various concentrations (Fig. 9.7). A dose-dependent effect appears to exist at concentrations between 10^{-8} and 10^{-5} M in the presence of a constant concentration of 10^{-5} M NA. This suggests that fluphenazine has a high affinity for the NA-sensitive

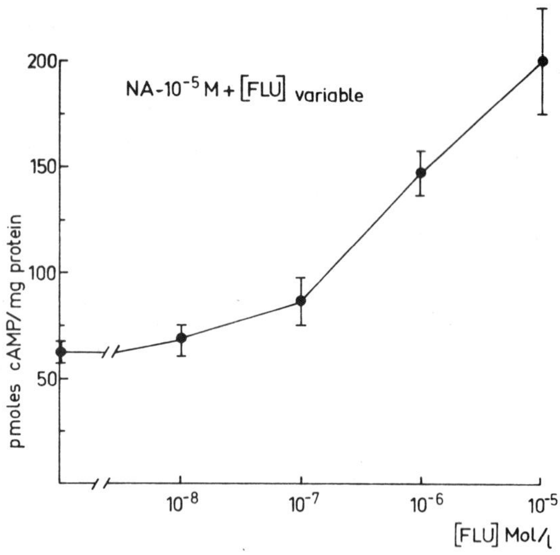

Fig. 9.7. Cyclic AMP levels in rat retina incubated with 10^{-5} M noradrenaline (NA) in the presence of various concentrations of fluphenazine (FLU). Control values with and without NA and fluphenazine: 22 pmoles cAMP/mg protein; with fluphenazine: 26 pmoles cAMP/mg protein; number of experiments for each point: 4. Vertical bars: 2x S.E.M.

cAMP-synthetizing system.

Greengard et al. (1972) have offered evidence for a DA-receptor localized at the postsynaptic region of the superior cervical ganglion. It is tempting to assume the existence of a similar system in the neuronal network of the retina. Several criteria have been tested in order to promote DA to the status of neurotransmitter in the retina. These criteria are: location in typical cells, release after light stimulation, synthesis and breakdown, evoked electrical activity after exogenous application. Thus DA is a serious neurotransmitter candidate in the retina. In line with the model of Greengard there is reason to localize the DA-receptor at a postsynaptic site, where it is linked with a cAMP-synthetizing system.

Our results with haloperidol and fluphenazine suggest, however, the need to be cautious in ascribing effects only to a postsynaptic involvement of these drugs in affecting the DA- or NA-induced cAMP-synthesis. Certain drugs have a presynaptic site of action in addition to a postsynaptic one. A DA-agonist like apomorphine increases the turnover rate of DA in cerebral tissue, whereas DA-antagonists like haloperidol and clozapine decrease this turnover (Andén et al., 1963; Da Prada and Pletscher, 1966; Laverty and Sharman, 1965; Nybäck and Sedvall, 1968 and 1970). These drugs presumably act directly on DA-receptors which are located presynaptically, the so-called autoreceptors (Aghajanian and Bunney, 1974; Kehr et al., 1972). In order to establish the possible existence of DA-autoreceptors in the retina, the influence of these drugs on levels of homovanillic acid have been investigated in retina and corpus striatum.

Albino rats are given intraperitoneal injections of the drugs and are sacrificed after fixed periods. Homovanillic acid levels are measured in extracts of whole eyes and of corpus striatum (Westerink and Korf, 1975). In agreement with results of other investigators, marked increases of the homovanillic acid levels are found after treatment with haloperidol and clozapine (Table 9.4). After administration of apomorphine the levels of homovanillic acid are reduced. These results suggest that DA-containing neurons from retina and corpus striatum respond similarly after administration of drugs as haloperidol, clozapine and apomorphine, either by increasing or decreasing homovanillic acid levels. These levels reflect the turnover rate of DA. This turnover rate may, at least partly, be regulated by presynaptically localized autoreceptors (Aghajanian and Bunney, 1974; Kehr et al., 1972). In view of these observations it seems that neuroleptics and apomorphine do not only influence the action of DA on adenyl cyclases, but also exert a direct effect on dopaminergic neurons. The presence of autoreceptors may complicate the interpretation of effects of these drugs on synaptic processes in general, and on postsynaptic processes specifically.

CONCLUDING REMARKS

We have tested the effects of potassium ions and of catecholamines on the cAMP-levels in the retinal network of the rat.

The responsiveness of the adenyl cyclases, activated by naturally occurring

Table 9.4. Effects of drugs affecting dopamine metabolism on levels of homovanillic acid in retina and corpus striatum of rat

			Retina		Corpus striatum	
			homovanillic acid		homovanillic acid	
Drug	Dose mg/kg b.w.	Time between i.p. injection and sacrifice	ng/eye	percentage of control value	ng/g wet wt.	percentage of control value
none	-	-	5.4 ± 0.3 (8)	100 ± 5	0.45 ± 0.2 (15)	100 ± 44
apomorphine	5	60 min.	3.4 ± 0.4 (7)	63 ± 7	0.17 ± 0.03 (5)	38 ± 7
clozapine	15	120 min.	6.6 ± 0.4 (9)	122 ± 7	1.02 ± 0.08 (7)	227 ± 18
haloperidol	1	120 min.	11.9 ± 0.5 (4)	220 ± 9	2.97 ± 0.27 (9)	660 ± 60

Mean values ± S.E.M. are given with the number of experiments in parentheses. All values are significantly different from controls ($p < 0.002$; two-tailed Student-t-test). Results from experiments by Westerink and Korf (1975 and unpublished observations).

substances like K^+ ions, DA and NA, appears to be very high, since maximal activity is obtained within 2 min.

The cAMP-increases induced by K^+ ions and ouabain are probably caused by depolarization of cell membranes. Such a depolarization may affect the membrane conformation, which would then activate the adenyl cyclase system.

It is not sure whether K^+ ions and DA exert their effects by a single mechanism. This point must be subject of further research. Considering the results obtained with haloperidol, other local anaesthetics might be useful agents in this respect.

Our results of experiments with fluphenazine and haloperidol do not allow us to decide whether one receptor sensitive for DA as well as for NA exists, or two receptors sensitive either for DA or for NA. In the experiments of Kebabian et al. (1972) on the DA-sensitive system in the caudate nucleus, haloperidol suppresses the DA-activated cAMP-response as well as the NA-activated one. Hence, they conclude that there exists one catecholamine receptor adenyl cyclase system activated by DA and by NA.

It should be kept in mind that comparison of our data, obtained with intact, incubated retina, with those obtained from studies with broken cell preparations (Brown and Makman, 1972; Kebabian, 1972; Makman and Brown, 1975) is not fully permitted. The complex interactions between several adenyl cyclases and catecholamine receptors, which probably exist in the *in vivo* situation, will be retained better in the intact, incubated retina than in homogenates.

The results of our studies with fluphenazine and haloperidol suggest that these substances are not simply antagonists of the DA-receptor, since they exert a synergistic effect on the NA-induced cAMP-increase. Interpretation of the results with these neuroleptic drugs is made more complex by the demonstration of DA-sensitive autoreceptors, which are localized presynaptically. These receptors appear to be sensitive for haloperidol as well.

In experiments with the α-adrenergic blocker phentolamine and the β-adrenergic blockers sotalol and propanolol, we find phentolamine and sotalol without any effect on the DA- and NA-induced cAMP-synthesis. Propanolol (10^{-5} M) suppresses only the NA ($5x10^{-5}$ M) induced cAMP-increase by 50%. These findings suggest that the DA- and NA-effects cannot simply be explained by assuming the existence of one adrenergic receptor specifically sensitive for DA (see also Ames and Pollen, 1969; Makman et al., 1975). Whether the effects of NA represent a physiological role for NA in the retinal network or not, is not clear at this moment.

The localization of DA in the retina, its neurochemical and neuropharmacological properties and the effects of this catecholamine on the bioelectrical behaviour of cellular elements in the retina suggest some tentative conclusions about the physiological role of dopamine in the excited retina.

ACKNOWLEDGEMENTS

The authors gratefully acknowledge the expert technical assistance of mr. H. Roelse and mrs. T. Wieringa-Meyer in these experiments. They also wish to thank Prof.Dr. W.G. Walter and Dr. F. Veringa (Dept. of Neurophysiology, this

University) and members of the Department of Pharmacology (this University) for critical discussions during the course of this study. The authors are indebted to miss G. Popken for assistance in the preparation of the manuscript, to miss T. Douma for bibliographical assistance, to mr. Th. Deddens and mr. B. Tebbes for preparation of the illustrations, to mr. J. Mast for development of instrumental devices, and to mr. A. Blaauwwiekel and mr. F. van der Heide for skilful experimental assistance.

The results of these studies have been presented in part at the Fifth International Meeting of the International Society for Neurochemistry, Barcelona, Spain, 1-5 September 1975 (Abstract 131).

REFERENCES

Aghajanian G.K., and Bunney B.S. (1974) Pre- and postsynaptic feedback mechanisms in central dopaminergic neurons. In: Frontiers of neurology and neuroscience research (P. Seeman and G.M. Brown, Eds.); pp 4-11; Univ. Toronto Press, Toronto

Ames III, A., and Gurian B.S. (1963) Effects of glucose and oxygen deprivation on function of isolated mammalian retina. J. Neurophysiol. 26, 617-634

Ames III, A., and Pollen D.A. (1969) Neurotransmission in central nervous tissue. J. Neurophysiol. 32, 424-442

Andén N.E., Roos B.E. and Werdinius B. (1964) Effects of chlorpromazine, haloperidol and reserpine on the levels of phenolic acids in rabbit corpus striatum. Life Sciences, 3, 149-158

Ascher P. (1972) Inhibitory and excitatory effects of dopamine on aplysia neurones. J. Physiol. 225, 173-209

Bitensky M.W., Miki N., Marcus F.R., and Keirns J. (1973) The role of cyclic nucleotides in visual excitation. Life Sciences, 13, 1451-1472

Bourke R.S. (1969) Studies of the development and subsequent reduction of swelling of mammalian cerebral cortex under isosmotic conditions in vitro. Exp. Brain Res. 8, 232-248

Bourke R.S., Nelson K.M., Naumann R.A., and Young O.M. (1970) Studies of the production and subsequent reduction of swelling in primate cerebral cortex under isosmotic conditions in vivo. Exp. Brain Res. 10, 427-446

Brown J.H., and Makman M.H. (1972) Stimulation by dopamine of adenylate cyclase in retinal homogenates and of adenosine 3':5'-cyclic monophosphate formation in intact retina. Proc. Nat. Acad. Sci. USA, 69, 539-543

Brown J.H., and Makman M.H. (1973) Influence of neuroleptic drugs and apomorphine on dopamine sensitive adenylate cyclase of retina. J. Neurochem. 21, 477-479

Bucher M.B., and Schorderet M. (1975) Dopamine- and apomorphine-sensitive adenylate cyclase in homogenates of rabbit retina. Naunyn-Schmiedeberg's Arch. Pharmacol. 288, 103-107

Bunney B.S., Walter J.R., Roth R.H., and Aghajanian G.K. (1973) Dopaminergic neurons: effect of antipsychotic drugs and amphetamine on single cell activity. J. Pharmacol. Exp. Therap. 185, 560-571

Cramer H., Johnson D.G., Hanbauer I., Silberstein S.D., and Kopin I.J. (1973) Accumulation of adenosine 3',5'-monophosphate induced by catecholamines in the rat superior cervical ganglion in vitro. Brain Res. 53, 97-104

Da Prada M., and Pletscher A. (1966) Acceleration of the cerebral dopamine turnover by chlorpromazine. Experientia, 22, 465-467

Dowling J.E., and Werblin F.S. (1969) Organization of retina of the mudpuppy, Necturus maculosus I Synaptic structure. J. Neurophysiol. 32, 315-338

Dubin M.W. (1974) Anatomy of the vertebrate retina. In: The Eye (H. Davson and L.T. Graham Jr., Eds.); Vol. 6; 227-254; Acad. Press. New York

Duke-Elder S., and Cook C. (1963) System of ophthalmology (S. Duke-Elder, Ed.); Vol. III; 82-124

Eccles J.C. (1964) The excitatory response of spinal neurons. In: Progress in Brain Research (J.C. Eccles and J.P. Schadé, Eds.); Vol. 12; 1-34; Elsevier Publ. Comp., Amsterdam

Ehinger B., and Falck B. (1971) Autoradiography of some suspected neurotransmitter substances GABA, glycine, glutamic acid, histamine, dopamine and L-dopa. Brain Res. 33, 157-172

Falck B., Hillarp N.Å., Thieme G., and Torp A. (1962) Fluorescence of catecholamines and related compounds condensed with formaldehyde. J. Histochem. Cytochem. 10, 348-354

Ferrendelli J.A., Kinscherf D.A., and Chang M.M. (1973) Comparison of the effects of biogenic amines on cyclic GMP and cyclic AMP levels in mouse cerebellum in vitro. Brain Res. 84, 63-73

Franck G. (1970) Echanges cationique au niveau des neurones et des cellules gliales du cerveau. Arch. Int. Physiol. Biochim. 78, 613-866

Graham Jr. L.T. (1974) Comparative aspects of neurotransmitters in the retina. In: The Eye (H. Davson and L.T. Graham Jr., Eds.); Vol. 6; 283-342; Acad. Press. New York.

Greengard P., McAfee D.A., and Kebabian J.W. (1972) On the mechanism of action of cyclic AMP and its role in synaptic transmission. In: Advances in Cyclic Nucleotide Research (P. Greengard and G.A. Robinson, Eds.); Vol. I; 337-355; Raven Press, New York and North Holland Publ. Comp., Amsterdam

Häggendal J., and Malmfors T. (1965) Identification and cellular localization of the catecholamines in the retina and the choroid of the rabbit. Acta Physiol. Scand. 64, 58-66

Hertz L. (1966) Neuroglial localization of potassium and sodium effects on respiration in brain. J. Neurochem. 13, 1373-1387

Hertz L. (1968) Potassium effects on ion transport in brain slices. J. Neurochem. 15, 1-16

Hertz L. (1973) Ion effects on metabolism in the adult mammalian brain in vitro; evidence of a potassium induced stimulation of active uptake of KCl into neuroglial cells. Fadl's Forlag A/S, Köbenhavn, Danmark, pp 73-94

Huang M., Shimizu H., and Daly J. (1971) Regulation of adenosine cyclic 3', 5'-phosphate formation in cerebral cortical slices. Mol. Pharmacol. 7, 155-162

Huang M., and Daly J.W. (1974) Interrelationships among the levels of ATP, adenosine and cyclic AMP in incubated slices of guinea-pig cerebral cortex: effects of depolarizing agents, psychotropic drugs and metabolic inhibitors. J. Neurochem. 23, 393-404

Kebabian J.W., Petzold G.L., and Greengard P. (1972) Dopamine sensitive adenylate cyclase in caudate nucleus of rat brain and its similarity to the "dopamine receptor". Proc. Nat. Acad. Sci. USA, 69, 2145-2149

Kehr W.A., Carlsson A., Lindqvist M., Magnusson T., and Atack C.Y. (1972) Evidence for a receptor-mediated feedback control of striated tyrosine hydroxylase activity. J. Pharm. Pharmacol. 24, 744-747

Kerkut, G.A., Brown, L.C. and Walker, R.J. (1969) Postsynaptic stimulation of the electrogenic sodium pump. Life Sciences 8, 297-300
Kramer, S.G. (1971) Dopamine: A retinal neurotransmitter. I. Retinal uptake, storage, and light-stimulated release of ^{3}H-dopamine in vivo. Invest. Ophthal. 10, 438-452
Kramer, S.G., Potts, A.M. and Mangnall, Y. (1971) Dopamine: A retinal neurotransmitter. II. Autoradiographic localization of ^{3}H-dopamine in the retina. Invest. Ophthal. 10, 617-624
Laverty, R. and Sharman, D.F. (1965). Modification by drugs of the metabolism of 3',4'-dihydroxyphenylethylamine, noradrenaline and 5-hydroxytryptamine in the brain. Brit. J. Pharmacol. 24, 759-772
Lund-Andersen, H. and Hertz, L. (1970) Effects of potassium and glutamate on swelling and on sodium and potassium content in brain cortex slices from adult rats. Exp. Brain Res. 11, 199-212
Makman, M.H., Brown, J.H. and Mishra, R.K. (1975) Cyclic AMP in retina and caudate nucleus: influence of dopamine and other agents. In: Advances in Cyclic Nucleotide Research (Eds. Drummond, G.I., Greengard, P. and Robinson, G.A.). Vol. 5, 661-679. Raven Press, New York and North Holland Publ. Comp., Amsterdam
Malmfors, T. (1963) Evidence of adrenergic neurons with synaptic terminals in the retina of rats demonstrated with fluorescence and electron microscopy. Acta Physiol. Scand. 58, 99-100
McAfee, D.A., Schorderet, M. and Greengard, P. (1971) Adenosine 3',5'-monophosphate in nervous tissue: Increase associated with synaptic transmission. Science 171, 1156-1158
Mishra, R.K., Gardner, E.L., Katzman, R. and Makman, M.H. (1975) Enhancement of dopamine-stimulated adenylate cyclase activity in rat caudate after lesions in substantia nigra: Evidence for denervation supersensitivity. Proc. Nat. Acad. Sci. USA 71, 3883-3887
Nichols, C.W., Jacobowitz, D. and Hottenstein, M. (1967) The influence of light and dark on the catecholamine content of the retina and choroid. Invest. Ophthal. 6, 642-646
Nybäck, H. and Sedvall, G. (1968) Effect of chlorpromazine on accumulation and disappearance of catecholamines formed from tyrosine-^{14}C in brain. J. Pharmacol. Exp. Therap. 162, 294-301
Nybäck, H. and Sedvall, G. (1970) Further studies on the accumulation and disappearance of catecholamines formed from ^{14}C-tyrosine in mouse brain; Effect of some phenothiazine analogues. Europ. J. Pharmacol. 10, 193-205
Roch, P. and Kalix, P. (1975) Adenosine 3',5'-monophosphate in bovine superior cervical ganglion: Effect of high extracellular potassium. Bioch. Pharmacol. 24, 1293-1296
Shepherd, G.M. (1974) The synaptic organization of the brain; Oxford University Press, New York, pp. 145-178
Stell, W.K. (1972) The morphological organization of the vertebrate retina. In: Handbook of Sensory Physiology; Physiology of photoreceptor organs (Ed. Fuortes, M.G.). Vol. VII/2, 112-213. Springer Verlag, Berlin
Straschill, M. and Perwein, J. (1969) The inhibition of retinal ganglion cells by catecholamines and γ-aminobutyric acid. Pflüger's Arch. 312, 45-54
Werblin, F.S. and Dowling, J.E. (1969) Organization of the retina of the mudpuppy, Necturus maculosus. II. Intracellular recording. J. Neurophysiol. 32, 339-355
Werblin, F.S. (1974) Organization of the vertebrate retina. In: The Eye (Eds. Davson, H. and Graham Jr., L.T.). Vol. 6, 257-281. Acad. Press, New York
Westerink, N.H.C. and Korf, J. (1975) Influence of drugs on striated and limbic homovanillic acid concentration in the rat brain. Europ. J. Pharmacol. 33, 31-40

CHAPTER 10

NEUROTRANSMITTERS AND THE ISOLATED OPTIC TRACT-SUPERIOR COLLICULUS OF THE GUINEA PIG

H. McIlwain

Department of Biochemistry, Institute of Psychiatry,
(British Postgraduate Medical Federation, University of London)
De Crespigny Park, Denmark Hill, London SE5 8AF, UK.

INTRODUCTION

The visual process includes transmission between the eye and the visual cortex and also other parts of the brain, and I am honoured to be accorded such extensive extra-retinal territory for the last brief contribution to this book.

One characteristic of extra-retinal components of the visual system, especially in mammals, is that they have been little studied biochemically in comparison with the retina. Contributing to this appears to be a reluctance on the part of investigators to examine isolated systems parallelling those so successfully used in retinal studies. I therefore begin by describing work which employs an isolated system comprising an optic tract, lateral geniculate and superior colliculus of the guinea pig. Subsequently I would like to consider a specific aspect of transmission *in vivo*. Choice of substances examined has followed from observations of a high content of γ-aminobutyrate in the superior colliculi; from effects of lysergic acid diethylamide on the visual system and its antagonism to serotonin; and from the occurrence of adenine mononucleotides as counter-ions to stored biogenic amines.

AN ISOLATED OPTIC TRACT-SUPERIOR COLLICULAR PREPARATION

This OT-SC preparation has been developed in Yamamoto's laboratory and in our own (Kawai & Yamamoto, 1967, 1969; Heller & McIlwain, 1973). Preparation in the guinea pig consists of opening the skull, and removing the brain with the optic nerves before they reach the chiasma. In the separated brain with its central surface uppermost, the chiasma is divided at its midline and one optic tract preserved, plus the brainstem to which it is fused; this carries the posterior hypothalamus, cerebral peduncle, lateral geniculate body and superior colliculus. The optic tract is cut from the preduncle with fine scissors, and the lower part of the peduncle cut away. With a bow-cutter and recessed glass guide (McIlwain, 1975) a slice of 0.35 - 0.4 mm is cut from the superior colliculus and lateral geniculate body keeping intact the connection to the optic tract. The whole weights about 15 mg and takes about 3 min. to prepare (see Fig. 10.1).

OUTPUT OF POSSIBLE NEUROHUMORAL AGENTS, AND RESPONSES TO THEM

In use, the OT-SC preparation is promptly transferred to a bicarbonate-glucose saline at 38^{0} in equilibrium with O_2-5% CO_2, contained in vessels suitable for superfusion or for electrophysiological work. In our own experiments (Heller & McIlwain, 1973) such preparations were superfused and stimulated electrically at the part of the optic tract distal from the colliculus. They were employed in experiments concerned with the possible role of adenine derivatives as neurohumoral agents in parts of the brain, and to this end the OT-SC preparation was preincubated in media which contained $[^{14}C]$adenine. Following preincubation the excess of ^{14}C was washed out by superfusion; electrical stimulation at the tract was then found to give increased output of ^{14}C, identified as being in the form of adenosine and a number of its derivatives. The time-course of output in one experiment is shown in Fig. 10.1; here, the tract was interrupted by cutting it, at about the level of the lateral geniculate. This left a small response only to stimulation; response was much greater when the stimulating pulses were applied to the tract beyond the cut, and nearer to the colliculus.

Note also that in these experiments the electrical stimulation increased the tissue's glycolysis. In the instance quoted, the increase caused in glycolysis parallelled that caused in the output of adenine derivatives, but circumstances have been found in which the two responses are dissociated. The status of adenosine as a neurohumoral agent in parts of the mammalian brain has received comment elsewhere (Burnstock, 1972; McIlwain, 1972, 1976; Krnjevic, 1974); the compound depresses evoked cell-firing or induced changes in potential, in cerebellar neurons or in the piriform cortex.

On stimulating the optic tract in similarly-isolated OT-SC preparations, Kawai (1970) found an increased output of serotonin. Sectioning the tract showed that the serotonin was coming from the colliculus and not from other parts of the system. This output was inhibited when bathing fluids contained 0.1 - 1 μM lysergic acid diethylamide. When serotonin was applied to a normal OT-SC preparation, it modified the cell-firing induced on the superior colliculus by stimulation at the optic tract (Kawai & Yamamoto, 1969). Stimulation ordinarily gave deflections judged to be the field potential of a postsynaptic response, and 0.1 - 1 μM serotonin progressively diminished the amplitude of

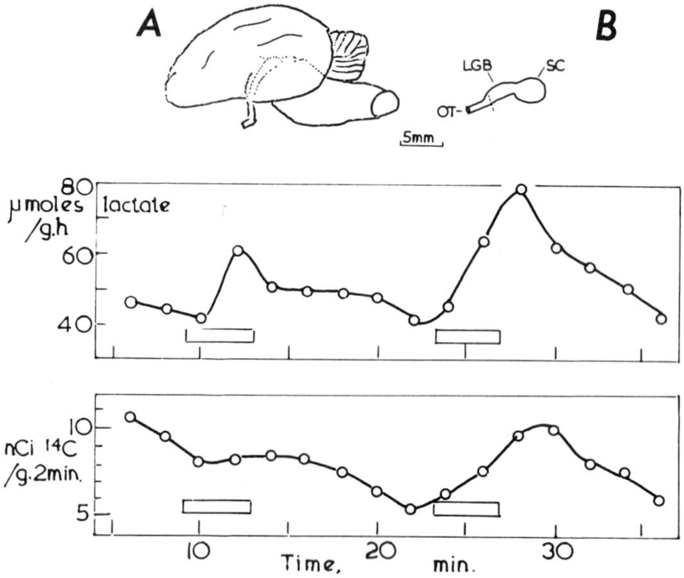

Fig. 10.1. The isolated optic tract-superior collicular system prepared from the guinea pig, and its response to excitation (Heller & McIlwain, 1973).

Above: A, the regions concerned, in situ in the freshly dissected brain; B, after preparation; OT, optic tract; LGB, lateral geniculate body; SC, superior colliculus; a dotted line indicates the position of a cut.

Centre: the output of lactate from the superfused isolated system, initially unstimulated; then for the 4 min. shown by the first horizontal bar, stimulated peripheral to the cut; then for the 4 min. shown by the second horizontal bar, stimulated central to the cut.

Below : the output of ^{14}C from $[^{14}C]$adenine concomitant with that of lactate described above.

the responses. Prior exposure of the tissue to 0.01 - 1 μM lysergic acid diethylamide potentiated or diminished the effect of serotonin; interactions were analysed in detail and depended on concentrations and times of exposure to the two agents. Lysergic acid diethylamide antagonizes serotonin in several biological systems, but this interaction in the optic system has especial relevance to the ability of the amide to induce visual hallucinations.

Sodium glutamate induced cell-firing in superior collicular neurons of the preparation, but such firing was not modified by serotonin (Kawai & Yamamoto, 1969). Noradrenaline and dopamine did not modify the serotonin action; lysergic acid ethylamide acted as did the diethylamide, and bufotenin had a lesser action. Using the isolated OT-SC preparation the normal responses at the superior colliculus to electrical stimulation of the optic tract were found to be diminished by 0.05 - 0.28 mM-γ-aminobutyrate (Kawai & Yamamoto, 1967). The aminobutyrate did not have comparable actions in similarly-handled tissues from the neocortex.

The inhibitory action of γ-aminobutyric acid in the OT-SC preparation of the guinea pig required the presence of chloride ions in incubating fluids, and the acid was concluded to act by increasing membrane permeability to the chloride ion. In this action, γ-aminobutyric acid mimicked the behaviour of the natural inhibitory transmitter of the superior colliculus (Kawai & Yamamoto, 1967).

A VECTORIAL ASPECT TO NEUROTRANSMITTER REUPTAKE

The aspect of transmission in visual systems *in vivo* to which I now turn concerns movement of materials by axonal flow. The substances so transported in many neural systems, include neurotransmitters and enzymes involved in their metabolism; trophic actions postsynaptically observed have long been recognized as prominent effects of substances axonally transported (see for example Ochs, 1965).

Part of the mechanism of such transport in the visual system has been displayed by the use of colchicine (Karlsson & Sjostrand, 1971 *a*, *b*). This binds to the microtubular protein which participates in axonal transport, the combination being demonstrated after labelling the microtubular protein of the optic nerve and tract of the rabbit by intraocular injection of $[^3H]$leucine. Following the blocking of flow, a failure in synaptic transmission was observed and concluded to be due to lack of transmission of materials from perikarya to nerve terminal (Rahmann & Breer, 1975).

Table 10.1. AXONAL TRANSPORT and OPTIC SYSTEMS

Species and injection	Substances administered	Route identified
1. Tegu lizard; intraocular	^{3}H Leucine, proline	Retina to lateral geniculate and mesencephalic tectum
2. Teleost; intraocular	^{3}H Leucine; N-Acetylmannosamine	Retina to optic tectum
3. Chick; intraocular	^{3}H Proline, fucose	Retina to optic tectum; includes glycoproteins
4. Chick; optic tectum	Horseradish peroxidase	Optic tectum to retina; in retinal ganglion cells; retrograde
5. Rabbit; intraocular	^{3}H Leucine	Retinal ganglion cells to lateral geniculate
6. Rabbit; striate cortex	^{3}H Adenosine, uridine	Striate to lateral geniculate; and lateral posterior thalamus
7. Ferret (rat, cat) intraocular	^{3}H Leucine	To superchiasmatic nucleus; anterior hypothalamus, contralateral

References: 1. Cruce & Cruce, 1975; 2. Rakmann & Breer, 1975; 3. Marchisio *et al.*, 1975; 4. La Vail & La Vail, 1975; 5. Karlsson & Sjöstrand, 1971 a, b; 6. Schubert & Kreutzberg, 1974; 7. Thorpe, 1975.

Examples of axonal transport in optic systems are listed in Table 10.1; note the popularity in such research of intraocular injection, which in several cases has been shown to involve uptake at the retina of materials which are subsequently detected, by autoradiography or by dissection and analyses, at the lateral geniculate or other regions within the brain. The transmission is, indeed, displayed at all levels of the optic system from retina to visual cortex, and in both orthograde and retrograde senses.

Of the investigations enumerated in Table 10.1, those concerning adenosine (Schubert & Kreutzberg, 1974) give data which valuably complement others which describe from neural systems an output of adenosine or its derivatives. Loss of ATP from a denervated muscle is an old observation (Ochs, 1965), and as you will recall from earlier data, we have found (Heller & McIlwain, 1973) appreciable output of adenosine derivatives from the OT-SC system, an output increased by stimulation. In preparations from other parts of the mammalian brain, we have shown (Kuroda & McIlwain, 1974) that a loss of adenosine derivatives occurs specifically from nerve terminals; that it is increased by excitation; and that the adenosine and its derivatives which appear extracellularly are subsequently taken up again by the tissue.

Now in the optic system of the rabbit, neural elements which participate in such uptake have been specified. Schubert & Kreutzberg (1974-5) have demonstrated by autoradiography a transfer of adenosine from nerve terminals to the postsynaptic cells which they innervate. Their observations, summarized in Table 10.2, indicate that $[^3H]$adenosine applied to the striate cortex is found there largely in the cell bodies as trichloroacetic acid-soluble compounds, and is transported axonally to the lateral geniculate. Little goes to the animals' general circulation, for the contralateral side of the geniculate acquires negligible ^3H. Some of the ^3H is probably as ribonucleic acid, but most appears to be transported as oligonucleotides and to arrive at the terminals of cortical neurons, and also postsynaptically at the cell bodies which they surround.

Processes which take up a neurotransmitter after its release are frequently seen as terminating its action, or as effecting economy by its reuse. The observations described give a vectorial character to the reuptake and emphasize its likely association with the trophic phenomena which are part of neural connectivity. A similar vectorial component in uptake and release of amino

Table 10.2 AXONAL MOVEMENT OF ^{3}H OF [^{3}H]ADENOSINE from striate cortex to lateral geniculate nucleus, rabbit. Schubert & Kreutzberg, 1974.

<u>Injected</u>: [^{3}H]adenosine, 66 nmoles in 10 μl

<u>Radioactivity observed</u> autoradiographically in samples <u>taken 1-3 days later</u>:

(I) At injection site, most in neuron cell-bodies

(II) In ipsilateral geniculate nucleus and fibre bundles leading there: increasing activities, 1-3 days

(III) TCA soluble material is 93% of whole; remainder insoluble in TCA and under histological fixation conditions

(IV) Actinomycin D at cortex diminished the ^{3}H "fixed" there but had little effect on the arrival of material at geniculate

(V) Transported activity corresponds to 25 μM adenosine; <1% of this found at contralateral side.

acids was pointed out previously (McIlwain, 1970; Jones & McIlwain, 1971); the release was diminished by colchicine. Output and reuptake of these essential metabolites - purines, amino acids and their precursors or products - can thus result in a net movement of the substances concerned into and out of the brain. Relevant movements can begin (Table 10.1) from the eye or from the cerebral cortex; the eye as portal to the mind transmits materials (not all of them orthodox neurotransmitters) as well as nerve impulses.

REFERENCES

Burnstock G. (1972) Purinergic nerves. Pharmacol. Rev. <u>24</u>, 509-581

Cruce W.L.R. & Cruce J.A.F. (1975) Projections from the retina to the lateral geniculate: a comparison of anterograde transport and anterograde degeneration. Brain Res. <u>85</u>, 221-228

Heller I.H. & McIlwain H (1973) Release of [^{14}C]adenine. Brain Research <u>53</u>, 105-116

Jones D.A. & McIlwain H. (1971) Amino acid production and translocation in incubated and superfused tissues from the brain. J. Neurobiol. <u>2</u>, 311-326

Karlsson J-O & Sjostrand J. (1971 <u>a</u>) Synthesis, migration and turnover of

protein in retinal ganglion cells. J. Neurochem. 18, 749-767
Karlsson J-O & Sjostrand J. (1971 b) Transport of microtubular protein in axons of retinal ganglion cells. J. Neurochem. 18, 975-892
Kawai N. (1970) Release of 5-hydroxytryptamine from slices of superior colliculus by optic tract stimulation. Neuropharmacology 9, 395-397
Kawai N. & Yamamoto C. (1967) Effects of γ-aminobutyric acid on the potentials evoked in vitro in the superior colliculus. Experientia 23, 822-823
Kawai N. & Yamamoto C. (1969) Effects of 5-hydroxytryptamine, LSD and related compounds on electrical activities evoked in vitro in thin slices from the superior colliculus. Int. J. Neuropharm. 8, 437-449
Krnjevic K. (1974) Chemical nature of synaptic transmission in vertebrates. Physiol. Rev. 54, 418-540
Kuroda & McIlwain H. (1974) Uptake and release $[^{14}C]$adenine derivatives at beds of mammalian cortical synaptosomes in a superfusion system. J. Neurochem. 22, 691-699
La Vail M. & La Vail J.H. (1975) Reterograde intraaxonal transport of horseradish peroxidase in retinal ganglion cells of the chick. Brain Res. 85, 273-280
Marchisio P.C., Gremo F. & Sjostrand J. (1975) Axonal transport in embryonic neurons. The possibility of a proximo-distal axolemmal transfer of glycoproteins. Brain Res. 85, 281-285
McIlwain H. (1970) Excitation and movement of materials on superfusing cerebral tissues. Wates Foundation Sympos. on the Blood-Brain Barrier, 85-91; Edit. R.V. Coxon. Oxford: Truex
McIlwain H. (1972) Regulatory significance of the release and action of adenine derivatives in cerebral systems. Biochem. Soc. Symp. 36, 69-85
McIlwain H. (1975) Practical Neurochemistry pp 105-121; 282-284 London: Churchill Livingstone
McIlwain H. (1976) Transport of adenine derivatives in tissues of the brain. ISN Sattelite Symposium, Transport Phenomena in the Nervous System Edit. Battistin & Lajtha. New York, Plenum
Ochs S. (1965) Elements of Neurophysiology, p. 147-152; 177-181. New York: Wiley.
Rahmann H. & Breer H. (1975) Neuronal transport of low molecular compounds in the CNS of releosts. Brain Res. 85, 301-305
Schubert P. & Kreutzberg G.W. (1974) Axonal transport of adenosine and uridine derivatives and transfer to postsynaptic neurons. Brain Res. 76, 526-530
Schubert P. & Kreutzberg G.W. (1975) $[^{3}H]$ Adenosine, a tracer for neuronal connectivity. Brain Res. 85, 317-319
Thorpe P.A. (1975) Presence of a retinohypothalamic projection in the ferret. Brain Res. 85, 343-346

INDEX

Fluphenazine, and DA-induced cAMP-synthesis, 209-213